Acute Coronary Syndrome: Urgent and Follow-up Care

The Cardiovascular Team Approach

A book series focusing on the interprofessional team approach
for the management and prevention of cardiovascular diseases.

Editors-in-Chief:
Joseph S. Alpert, MD, FAHA, FACC, MACP, FESC
Lynne T. Braun, PhD, CNP, FAHA, FPCNA, FAANP, FAAN
Barbara J. Fletcher, RN, MN, FAHA, FAAN
Gerald Fletcher, MD, FAHA, FACC, FACP

Look for these and other forthcoming series titles from
Cardiotext Publishing.

Volume 1: *Heart Failure: Strategies to Improve Outcomes*
Ileana L. Piña, MD, MPH, FACC, FAHA, and
Elizabeth A. Madigan, PhD, RN, FAAN, editors

Volume 2: *Prehospital Management of Acute STEMI: Practical Approaches and International Strategies for Early Intervention*
Edgardo Escobar, MD, FACC, FAHA, and
Alejandro Barbagelata, MD, FAHA, FSCAI, editors

Volume 3: *Acute Coronary Syndrome: Urgent and Follow-up Care*
Eileen Handberg, PhD, ARNP-BC, FAHA, FACC, and
R. David Anderson, MD, MS, FACC, FSCAI, editors

Volume 4: *Atrial Fibrillation: A Multidisciplinary Approach to Improving Patient Outcomes*
N.A. Mark Estes III, MD, FACC, FHRS, FAHA, FESC, and
Albert L. Waldo, MD, PhD (Hon), FACC, FHRS, FAHA, FACCP, editors

Please visit www.cardiotextpublishing.com for more information about this series.

Acute Coronary Syndrome: Urgent and Follow-up Care

The Cardiovascular Team Approach Series

VOLUME 3

Eileen Handberg, PhD, ARNP-BC, FAHA, FACC
R. David Anderson, MD, MS, FACC, FCSAI
Volume Editors

Joseph S. Alpert, MD, FAHA, FACC, MACP, FESC
Lynne T. Braun, PhD, CNP, FAHA, FPCNA, FAANP, FAAN
Barbara J. Fletcher, RN, MN, FAHA, FAAN
Gerald Fletcher, MD, FAHA, FACC, FACP
Editors-in-Chief

cardiotext.
PUBLISHING
Minneapolis, Minnesota

Cardiotext Publishing, LLC
3405 W. 44th Street
Minneapolis, Minnesota 55410
USA

www.cardiotextpublishing.com

Any updates to this book may be found at: www.cardiotextpublishing.com/acute-coronary-syndrome-urgent-and-follow-up-care

Comments, inquiries, and requests for bulk sales can be directed to the publisher at: info@cardiotextpublishing.com.

Library of Congress Control Number: 2017930918

ISBN: 978-1-935395-94-2

eISBN: 978-1-935395-38-6

Printed in the United States of America

Contents

About the Editors-in-Chief

Editors-in-Chief

Joseph S. Alpert, MD, FAHA, FACC, MACP, FESC
Professor of Medicine, University of Arizona Health Science Network; Editor-in-Chief, *The American Journal of Medicine*, Tucson, Arizona

Lynne T. Braun, PhD, CNP, FAHA, FPCNA, FAANP, FAAN
Professor, Department of Adult Health and Gerontological Nursing, Rush University College of Nursing; Nurse Practitioner, Division of Cardiology, Rush University Medical Center, Chicago, Illinois

Barbara J. Fletcher, RN, MN, FAHA, FAAN
Clinical Associate Professor, Brooks College of Health, School of Nursing, University of North Florida, Jacksonville, Florida

Gerald Fletcher, MD, FAHA, FACC, FACP
Professor in Medicine (Cardiovascular Diseases), Mayo Clinic College of Medicine, Mayo Clinic Florida, Jacksonville, Florida

About the Authors

Editors

Eileen Handberg, PhD, ARNP-BC, FAHA, FACC
Research Professor of Medicine, Director, Clinical Trials Program, Division of Cardiovascular Medicine, College of Medicine, University of Florida, Gainesville, Florida

R. David Anderson, MD, MS, FACC, FCSAI
Professor of Medicine, Director of Interventional Cardiology, Division of Cardiovascular Medicine, College of Medicine, University of Florida, Gainesville, Florida

Contributors

Brandon Allen, MD
Assistant Professor, Department of Emergency Medicine, College of Medicine, University of Florida, Gainesville, Florida

Staccie A. Allen, MSN, ARNP, EMT-P, CFRN
Program Director, ShandsCair Flight Program, Department of Emergency Medicine, College of Medicine, University of Florida, Gainesville, Florida

Anthony A. Bavry, MD, MPH
Associate Professor of Medicine, Division of Cardiovascular Medicine, College of Medicine, University of Florida, Gainesville, Florida; North Florida/South Georgia Veterans Health System, Malcom Randall VA Medical Center, Gainesville, Florida

Kathy Berra, MSN, ANP-BC, FAANP, FPCNA, FAAN
Co-Director, The LifeCare Company; Cardiovascular Medicine and Coronary Interventions, Redwood City, California; Nurse Practitioner Emeritus, Stanford Prevention Research Center, Stanford University School of Medicine, Palo Alto, California

Garrett Brown, MD
Cardiovascular Medicine Fellow, Division of Cardiovascular Medicine, College of Medicine, University of Florida, Gainesville, Florida

Calvin Choi, MD, MS
Assistant Professor of Medicine, Division of Cardiovascular Medicine, University of Florida, Gainesville, Florida; North Florida/South Georgia Veterans Health System, Malcom Randall VA Medical Center, Gainesville, Florida

Andrew M. Freeman, MD, FACC, FACP
Director, Cardiovascular Prevention and Wellness; Director of Clinical Cardiology; Associate Professor of Medicine, Division of Cardiology, National Jewish Health, Denver, Colorado

Ty J. Gluckman, MD, FACC, FAHA
Medical Director, Clinical Transformation, Providence Heart and Vascular Institute, Providence St. Vincent Medical Center, Portland, Oregon

Preeti Jois, MD, FACEP
Medical Director, Humana, Central Florida; Founder/CEO Jois MD Consulting LLC; Assistant Professor, Emergency Medicine, UCF College of Medicine; Capt, USAFR, MC, CCATT, Patrick AFB, Florida

Jason Jones, MD
Clinical Assistant Professor, Department of Emergency Medicine, College of Medicine, University of Florida, Gainesville, Florida

Dharam J. Kumbhani, MD, SM, MRCP, FACC, FAHA, FSCAI
Assistant Professor of Medicine, Interventional Cardiologist, Department of Internal Medicine, University of Texas Southwestern Medical School, Dallas, Texas

Samantha Noah, RN
Emergency Medicine, North Florida/South Georgia Veterans Health System, Malcom Randall VA Medical Center, Gainesville, Florida

Andre R. M. Paixao, MD
Cardiologist, Arkansas Heart Hospital, Little Rock, Arkansas

Ki Park, MD
Assistant Professor of Medicine, Division of Cardiovascular Medicine, College of Medicine, University of Florida, Gainesville, Florida; North Florida/South Georgia Veterans Health System, Malcom Randall VA Medical Center, Gainesville, Florida

Joel Rowe, MD
EMS Fellow, Department of Emergency Medicine, College of Medicine, University of Florida, Gainesville, Florida

Garrett Ruth, MD
Cardiovascular Medicine Fellow, Division of Cardiovascular Medicine, College of Medicine, University of Florida, Gainesville, Florida

Robert S. Svingos, PharmD
Clinical Pharmacist/Emergency Department, North Florida/South Georgia Veterans Health System, Malcom Randall VA Medical Center, Gainesville, Florida; Clinical Assistant Professor, Pharmacotherapy and Translational Research, College of Pharmacy, University of Florida, Gainesville, Florida

Christine Van Dillen, MD
Assistant Professor, Department of Emergency Medicine, College of Medicine, University of Florida, Gainesville, Florida

Preface

Acute Coronary Syndrome: Urgent and Follow-up Care is a must-read for all those involved in the care of ACS, including EMS, nurses, advanced practice providers as well as physicians. This volume not only reviews the causes of ACS, but also provides evidence-based acute and follow-up treatment recommendations that incorporate the perspectives of all those involved in the care of these patients.

An example of successful team-based care in treating ACS patients is the reduction in time to treatment of STEMI patients, achieving door-to-balloon times well below 90 minutes. This process begins with EMS and incorporates the emergency department in the prompt diagnostic strategy that has resulted in rapid transit of the ACS patient to the catheterization laboratory for reperfusion therapy. The process continues with strategies for long-term secondary prevention that bring together social workers, nurses, physician assistants, nurse practitioners, and physicians in transitioning patients to home. This book provides a team-focused perspective to provide updated ACS treatment recommendations across the spectrum of disease.

The participation of all members of the healthcare system in ACS care is vital to program success, and this book highlights the role of the team in carrying out successful, guideline-driven care.

Abbreviations

AACVPR	American Association of Cardiovascular and Pulmonary Rehabilitation
ABC	airway, breathing, and circulation
ABIM	American Board of Internal Medicine
ACC	American College of Cardiology
ACE	angiotensin-converting enzyme
ACEP	American College of Emergency Physician
ACS	acute coronary syndrome
ADP	adenosine diphosphate
AED	automatic external defibrillator
AHA	American Heart Association
AHRQ	Agency for Healthcare Research and Quality
AMI	acute myocardial infarction
aPTT	activated partial thromboplastin time
ARB	angiotensin receptor blocker
ASCVD	atherosclerotic cardiovascular disease
BB	beta blocker
BMI	body mass index
CABG	coronary artery bypass graft
CAD	computer-aided dispatch
CAD	coronary artery disease
CCB	calcium-channel blocker
CDC	Centers for Disease Control
CHD	coronary heart disease
CHF	congestive heart failure
CI	confidence interval

CV	cardiovascular
CVD	cardiovascular disease
D2B	door-to-balloon
DALYs	disability-adjusted life years
DM	diabetes mellitus
ED	emergency department
ELSA	English Longitudinal Study of Aging
EMS	emergency medical service
EMT	emergency medical technician
ESC	European Society of Cardiology
HCP	healthcare provider
HDL	high-density lipoprotein
HIT	heparin-induced thrombocytopenia
HRS	Health Retirement Survey
HTN	hypertension
ICS	intercostal space
IV	intravenous
IVUS	intravascular ultrasound
LAD	left anterior descending
LBBB	left bundle branch block
LDL	low-density lipoprotein
LOE	level of evidence
LVEF	left ventricular ejection fraction
MACE	major adverse cardiac events
MI	myocardial infarction
MVD	microvascular dysfunction
NCDs	noncommunicable diseases
NHANES	National Health and Nutrition Examination Survey
NSTE-ACS	non-ST elevation ACS
NSTEMI	non-ST-segment elevation myocardial infarction
PCI	percutaneous coronary intervention
RAAS	renin-angiotensin-aldosterone system
RITA	Randomized Intervention Trial of Unstable Angina
RR	relative risk
RV	right ventricle
SCAD	spontaneous coronary artery dissection
SHARE	Survey of Health, Ageing, and Retirement

SL	sublingual
STEMI	ST-segment elevation myocardial infarction
SUTTP	Stepping up to the Plate
TOS	The Obesity Society
UA	unstable angina
UFH	unfractionated heparin
URL	upper reference limit
vIVUS	virtual histology intravascular ultrasound (or virtual IVUS)
VKA	vitamin K antagonists
VSD	ventricular septal defect
VSR	ventricular septal rupture
WHF	World Heart Federation

CHAPTER 1

Epidemiology

Garrett Ruth, MD, Garrett Brown, MD, Eileen Handberg, PhD, ARNP-BC, and R. David Anderson, MD, MS

INTRODUCTION

Acute coronary syndrome (ACS) is a term used for any condition brought on by sudden, reduced blood flow to the heart. The diagnosis of an ACS includes a spectrum of disease presentation ranging from unstable angina, to non-ST-segment elevation myocardial infarction (MI), to ST-segment elevation MI. It is usually associated with coronary artery disease (CAD), most commonly atherosclerosis. All of these conditions can progress to advancing disease and eventually lead to death. In many developed countries, heart disease is the leading cause of morbidity and mortality. Although the overall mortality rate in the United States has declined, CAD claims more than one-third of the deaths in persons over 35 years of age. Population data have shown that 1 of 2 men and 1 of 3 women in the United States will present with some symptomatic CAD in their lifetime. As the population gets older, the prevalence of CAD steadily increases. The 2010 Heart Disease and Stroke Statistics review reported that 17.6 million people in the United States have CAD.[1]

CARDIOVASCULAR DISEASE RISK FACTORS

CAD is localized to the heart but is a part of a larger group of atherosclerotic diseases classified as cardiovascular disease.

Acute Coronary Syndrome: Urgent and Follow-up Care © 2017
Joseph S. Alpert, Lynne T. Braun, Barbara J. Fletcher, Gerald Fletcher, Editors-in-Chief,
Cardiotext Publishing, ISBN: 978-1-935395-94-2

Cardiovascular disease refers to atherosclerosis that affects the entire arterial circulation, not just the coronary arteries. There are many manifestations including stroke, transient ischemic attack, angina, MI, and claudication. Cardiovascular disease is present in various populations but has an increased incidence in groups with specific risk factors. A growing trend of comorbidities such as obesity, hypertension, tobacco use, and cholesterol levels all contribute to the increasing overall burden of cardiovascular disease.

The prevalence of **obesity** (body mass index [BMI] ≥30 kg/m^2) has doubled in the years 1980 to 2008, and over 2.8 million deaths per year are attributed to being overweight (BMI ≥25 kg/m^2) or obese. In 1980, population statistics showed 5% of men and 8% of women were classified as obese. In 2008, 10% of men and 14% of women across the world were considered obese. It has also been shown that America has the highest prevalence of overweight (62%) and obese (26%) individuals (**Figure 1.1**).[2]

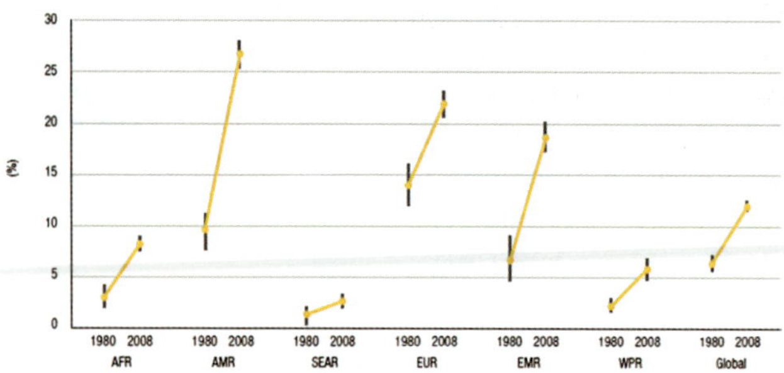

Figure 1.1

Change over time in mean BMI by WHO region, 1980 to 2008.

AFR = African region; AMR = Americas region; BMI = body mass index; EMR = Eastern Mediterranean region; EUR = European region; SEAR = South-East Asia region; WPR = West Pacific region. (*Source:* Reprinted with permission from World Health Organization. World Health Statistics. 2012.)

Population studies have shown that, worldwide, 40% of people older than age 25 have **hypertension**, and the number of people with elevated blood pressure has increased from 600 million in 1980 to a billion in 2008. This number will continue to grow and has been estimated to be 1.6 billion by the year 2025. Elevated blood pressure not only contributes to cardiovascular deaths (45%) but also has been found to be a contributing factor to more than 51% of stroke deaths worldwide.

Mean cholesterol levels have improved globally since the 1980s with the advent of statins, but still remain elevated in some developed countries. These decreases have been shown to be most significant in the high-income countries (mean decrease from 5.62 to 5.19 mmol/L) compared with low-income countries (4.46–4.20 mmol/L) and middle-income countries (4.91–4.7 mmol/L). Despite these improvements, 39% of the world's population has elevated cholesterol, with percentages >50% in some higher-income countries.

Smoking and **tobacco use** in the United States have declined over the past 25 years. Whereas in 1965 >40% of the population smoked, in 2010, this has decreased to 19.3%.[2] This is the fourth lowest rate of tobacco use among the countries involved in the Organization for Economic Cooperation and Development, behind Iceland, Sweden, and Mexico. From the most recent data, countries that still have >25% of residents who smoke include Greece, Ireland, Hungary, Estonia, Spain, and Turkey.[3]

EPIDEMIOLOGY OF CORONARY ARTERY DISEASE

In a 2009 report that used National Health and Nutrition Examination Survey (NHANES) data, prevalence of MI was compared by gender in individuals of middle age (35–54 years) from the periods 1988 to 1994 and 1999 to 2004.[4] Overall, both studied periods demonstrated greater prevalence in men.

However, the trend showed a decrease in men (2.5–0.7 from 1988 to 1994 and 2.2–1.0 from 1999 to 2004) and an increase in women. The NHANES report noted that data were self-reported for MI and angina and likely underestimated the actual prevalence of advanced heart disease.

Two large postmortem studies have shown a reduction in the incidence of anatomic coronary heart disease (CHD) over time. In one particular report, over 2500 autopsies were performed from the years 1979 to 1994 recording the prevalence of clinical anatomic CHD. The patients were aged 20 to 60 years, and results showed a decrease from 42% to 32% in men and 29% to 16% in women when the specific periods 1979 to 1983 and 1990 to 1994 were compared.[5] However, in ages >60 years, there was no change in prevalence. In another study, over 3800 autopsies were performed on U.S. military personnel who died of combat or unintentional injuries in a 10-year span from 2001 to 2011. This particular cohort had an average age of 26 years and comprised 98% men. Results showed that CHD only was present in 8.5% of subjects.[6] This was a drastic difference in those studied in previous wartime years such as the Korean War in the 1950s (77%) and the Vietnam War in the 1960s (45%).

Using the Framingham study, both initial subjects and offspring have been studied, allowing recording of statistics in relation to CAD and events detailing both recognized and silent MI, angina pectoris, unstable angina, and sudden cardiac death.[7–9] From these data, the following conclusions were made:

a) In people at age 40, the lifetime risk of developing CAD is 49% in men and 32% in women. For those who reach age 70, the lifetime risk is 35% in men and 24% in women.
b) The incidence of total coronary disease rises with age; however, women lag behind men by 10 years. Related to more serious outcomes such as sudden cardiac death

and severe CAD, women lag behind by over 20 years, but these differences begin to attenuate with advancing age.[7] For example, comparing subjects aged 35 to 64 years with those aged 65 to 94 years, the incidence of CAD doubles in men and triples in women.

c) In the premenopausal population, extensive coronary disease and sudden cardiac death are rare. However, following menopause, the incidence and severity of coronary disease increases, with a threefold risk compared with women of the same age who are premenopausal, owing to the cardioprotective effects of estrogen.[7]

d) In the population below 65 years of age, the annual incidence of all coronary events in men (12 per 1000) more than equals the rate of all other atherosclerotic cardiovascular events combined (7 per 1000); in women, it equals the rate of the other events (5 per 1000). Beyond 65 years of age, coronary disease still predominates. Coronary events comprise 33% to 65% of atherosclerotic cardiovascular events in men and 28% to 58% in women.

e) In women under age 75 years, the initial symptom of coronary disease is more likely to be angina pectoris than MI.[8] Men typically have angina following MI (66%), while women who have angina have relatively uncomplicated disease or stable angina. MI includes a large portion of men in whom only 20% of infarctions are preceded by long-standing angina. If the infarction is silent, that number decreases even further.[8,9]

f) With the addition of medications for atherosclerotic disease such as statins and beta blockers the initial presentation of CHD has since changed. A case control study of adults with their initial event of coronary disease with acute MI ($n = 486$) or stable angina ($n = 916$) demonstrated that recent medical therapy has an effect on the clinical presentation.[10]

DECREASING PREVALENCE OF CAD

Two reports illustrate the decreasing incidence of CAD over time in developed countries. An analysis from the NHANES I Epidemiologic Follow-up study compared two cohorts of subjects, from 1971 to 1982 (10,869 patients) and from 1982 to 1992 (9774 patients).[11] The incidence of CAD decreased from 133 to 114 cases per 10,000 persons per year of follow-up. An even larger decline was seen in cardiovascular disease overall (from 294 to 225 cases per 10,000 persons per year).

A report from the Mayo Clinic examined the incidence of CHD over time in Olmsted County, Minnesota.[12] During the interval from 1979 to 1998, there was a declining trend in the age-adjusted incidence of any new coronary disease (MI, sudden death, unstable angina, or angiographically diagnosed CHD) from 57 to 50 cases per 10,000 persons (relative risk 0.91, 95% CI 0.82–1.01).

When including men, women, African Americans, and Caucasians, the mortality rate for all cardiovascular disease has decreased by over 25% since 1975. These rates were steadily declining but have since slowed starting around the 1990s.[1,9,13–22] The 2010 Heart Disease and Stroke Statistics update of the American Heart Association reported that from 1996 to 2006, death rates from cardiovascular disease declined about 29% leading to reductions in the incidence of CAD and mortality rate for both sudden and nonsudden cardiac death.[1]

The National Institutes of Health, National Heart, Lung and Blood Institute reported that the age-adjusted mortality rate for cardiovascular disease decreased from 543.7 per 100,000 in 1980 to 244.8 per 100,000 in 2008. **Figure 1.2** displays the decline of age-adjusted mortality rates from 1980 to 2008 for cardiovascular disease, CHD, and stroke.[1,9]

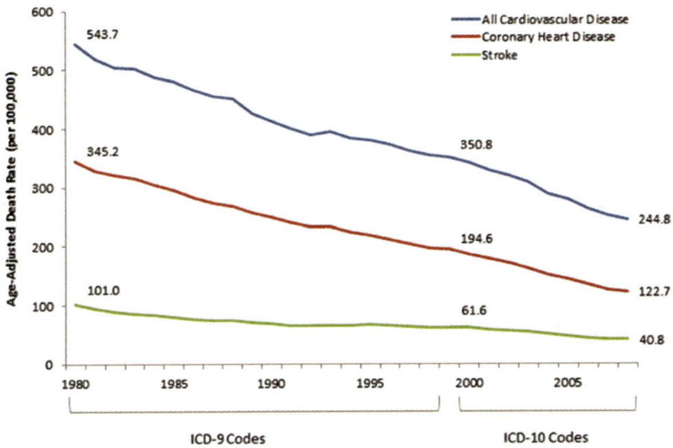

Figure 1.2

Age-adjusted death rates for cardiovascular disease, coronary heart disease, and stroke, 1980 to 2008. **Blue line** = all cardiovascular disease; **red line** = coronary heart disease; and **green line** = stroke. ICD = International Classification of Diseases. (*Source:* National Institutes of Health, National Heart, Lung and Blood Institute. Morbidity and Mortality: 2012 Chart Book on Cardiovascular, Lung, and Blood Diseases. [Public domain source].)

WORLDWIDE IMPACT OF CARDIOVASCULAR DISEASE

Cardiovascular disease (CVD) currently accounts for almost half of all noncommunicable diseases (NCDs). NCDs have surpassed communicable diseases (examples such as HIV/AIDS, tuberculosis, hepatitis, and sexually transmitted disease) with cardiovascular disease being the leading cause of death. Statistics currently show that CVD alone leads to more than 17 million deaths per year. With increasing population size, this estimate will grow to more than 23 million by 2030.[23,24] In specific populations, the majority of cardiovascular death occurs in the low- to middle-income countries, accounting for nearly 80% of total deaths globally. In higher-income countries, age tends to be much lower, and the incidence is greater in those areas where resources to address these issues are limited.[25, 26]

From 2011 to 2025, the projected economic loss from noncommunicable diseases is estimated to be $7.28 trillion. Approximately half of this amount represents CVD costs.[26] In comparison, if resources were spent on primary prevention of CVD and disease burden was decreased by 10%, this would lead to an estimated $377 billion reduction in total economic losses.[27] It has also been estimated that the cost of not investing in long-term prevention and further research into treatment of CVD could amount to as much as $47 trillion worldwide over the next 25 years. The World Health Organization has proposed "best buy" interventions in an effort to decrease the cost of worldwide NCDs. With the institution of these preventative measures for CVD (costing around $11–$13 billion dollars a year), this loss could be potentially avoided.[28] As stated previously, the low- to middle-income classes in developed countries will face the worst consequences, as this is where the majority of cardiovascular deaths occur.[29]

Disability-adjusted life years (DALYs) is a measure of disease burden related to the number of years lost due to disability or death from a given medical condition and the implications this has on a country as a whole. This can also relate to the caregiver who may have to cease work in order to take care of their family member. CVD is responsible for 10% of the DALYs lost in low- and middle-income countries, and 18% of DALYs lost in high-income countries.[30] This economic loss has major impacts on the developing world where cardiovascular disease affects a large percentage of able-bodied adults affected with CVD.[31]

HEART DISEASE AND STROKE BY COUNTRY

Population surveys across multiple developed nations assess the health and disease states of aging societies, including Survey of Health, Ageing, and Retirement (SHARE) in Europe and Health Retirement Survey (HRS), and English Longitudinal Study of Aging (ELSA) in the United States.[32] **Table 1.1** depicts data comparing age-adjusted prevalence of heart disease and stroke by country and shows that the United States exceeds other developed nations in prevalence of heart disease, with stroke ranking among the highest as well.[2]

Despite advancements in the diagnosis, treatment, and prevention of cardiovascular disease, it remains one of the

Table 1.1
Age-Adjusted Prevalence (% of Population) of Heart Disease and Stroke by Sex, 2004

Country	Heart Disease		Stroke	
	Males	Females	Males	Females
Austria	12.2	7.3	5.2	3.5
Belgium	18.8	11.8	3.9	4.2
Denmark	10.8	7.6	6.5	4.6
France	19.3	9.8	3.7	3.5
Germany	14.3	9.3	5.6	3.1
Greece	14.9	10.7	4.1	3.5
Italy	12.7	9.1	3.8	2.5
Netherlands	14.7	8.9	5.0	4.8
Spain	11.4	10.0	2.4	1.8
Sweden	20.3	13.0	6.3	3.6
Switzerland	9.5	5.4	2.9	2.2
Total SHARE	15.4	9.9	4.5	3.5
United States (HRS)	26.4	19.7	6.6	5.5
England (ELSA)	19.0	16.0	3.2	2.5

HRS = Health Retirement Survey; SHARE = Survey of Health, Ageing, and Retirement; ELSA = English Longitudinal Study of Aging. (*Source:* Reprinted from Laslett et al.[2] [STM publisher].)

world's most significant health concerns. With continued population growth, mortality rates may continue to increase especially in low-income countries, while they are decreasing in more developed nations. Research suggests that using preventative measures such as early diagnosis and broader use of established medical therapies, there has been a decrease in morbidity and mortality in certain populations. Many modifiable risk factors have been identified in population studies which, when addressed, have translated into improvements into age-adjusted incidences of heart disease and stroke. It is evident through these epidemiologic studies that cardiovascular disease as a whole will have a significant impact on global health and economy in the future.

REFERENCES

1. Lloyd-Jones D, Adams RJ, Brown TM, et al. Executive summary: heart disease and stroke statistics—2010 update: A report from the American Heart Association. *Circulation.* 2010;121:948–954.
2. Laslett LJ, Alagona P Jr, Clark BA 3rd, et al. The worldwide environment of cardiovascular disease: Prevalence, diagnosis, therapy, and policy issues. *J Am Coll Cardiol.* 2012;60(25 Suppl):S1–49.
3. OECD (2015). Tobacco consumption among adults, in *Health at a Glance 2015: OECD Indicators*, OECD Publishing, Paris. http://dx.doi.org/10.1787/health_glance-2015-en Accessed June 02, 2016.
4. Towfighi A, Zheng L, Ovbiagele B. Sex-specific trends in midlife coronary heart disease risk and prevalence. *Arch Intern Med.* 2009; 169:1762–6.
5. Roger VL, Weston SA, Killian JM, et al. Time trends in the prevalence of atherosclerosis: A population-based autopsy study. *Am J Med.* 2001;110:267–73.
6. Webber BJ, Seguin PG, Burnett DG, Clark LL, Otto JL. Prevalence of and risk factors for autopsy-determined atherosclerosis among U.S. service members, 2001–2011. *JAMA.* 2012;308:2577–2583.
7. Gordon T, Kannel WB, Hjortland MC, McNamara PM. Menopause and coronary heart disease. The Framingham Study. *Ann Intern Med.* 1978;89:157–161.
8. Lerner DJ, Kannel WB. Patterns of coronary heart disease morbidity and mortality in the sexes: A 26-year follow-up of the Framingham population. *Am Heart J.* 1986;111:383–390.

9. Kannel WB. Prevalence and clinical aspects of unrecognized myocardial infarction and sudden unexpected death. *Circulation.* 1987; 75(3 Pt 2):II4–5.
10. Go AS, Iribarren C, Chandra M, et al. Atherosclerotic Disease, Vascular Function and Genetic Epidemiology (ADVANCE) Study. Statin and beta-blocker therapy and the initial presentation of coronary heart disease. *Ann Intern Med.* 2006;144:229–238.
11. Ergin A, Muntner P, Sherwin R, He J. Secular trends in cardiovascular disease mortality, incidence, and case fatality rates in adults in the United States. *Am J Med.* 2004;117:219–227.
12. Arciero TJ, Jacobsen SJ, Reeder GS, et al. Temporal trends in the incidence of coronary disease. *Am J Med.* 2004;117:228–233.
13. Roger VL, Weston SA, Gerber Y, et al. Trends in incidence, severity, and outcome of hospitalized myocardial infarction. *Circulation.* 2010;121:863–869.
14. Parikh NI, Gona P, Larson MG, et al. Long-term trends in myocardial infarction incidence and case fatality in the National Heart, Lung, and Blood Institute's Framingham Heart study. *Circulation.* 2009;119:1203–1210.
15. Kuulasmaa K, Tunstall-Pedoe H, Dobson A, et al. Estimation of contribution of changes in classic risk factors to trends in coronary-event rates across the WHO MONICA Project populations. *Lancet.* 2000;355:675–687.
16. McGovern PG, Pankow JS, Shahar E, et al. Recent trends in acute coronary heart disease—mortality, morbidity, medical care, and risk factors. The Minnesota Heart Survey Investigators. *N Engl J Med.* 1996;334:884–890.
17. Capewell S, Morrison CE, McMurray JJ. Contribution of modern cardiovascular treatment and risk factor changes to the decline in coronary heart disease mortality in Scotland between 1975 and 1994. *Heart.* 1999;81:380–386.
18. Capewell S, Beaglehole R, Seddon M, McMurray J. Explanation for the decline in coronary heart disease mortality rates in Auckland, New Zealand, between 1982 and 1993. *Circulation.* 2000;102:1511–1516.
19. Cooper R, Cutler J, Desvigne-Nickens P, et al. Trends and disparities in coronary heart disease, stroke, and other cardiovascular diseases in the United States: Findings of the national conference on cardiovascular disease prevention. *Circulation.* 2000;102:3137–3147.
20. McGovern PG, Jacobs DR Jr, Shahar E, et al. Trends in acute coronary heart disease mortality, morbidity, and medical care from 1985 through 1997: The Minnesota heart survey. *Circulation.* 2001; 104:19–24.
21. Rosamond WD, Chambless LE, Folsom AR, et al. Trends in the incidence of myocardial infarction and in mortality due to coronary heart disease, 1987 to 1994. *N Engl J Med.* 1998;339:861–867.

22. Ford ES, Ajani UA, Croft JB, et al. Explaining the decrease in U.S. deaths from coronary disease, 1980–2000. *N Engl J Med.* 2007; 356:2388–2398.
23. World Health Organization. Cardiovascular Disease: Global Atlas on Cardiovascular Disease Prevention and Control. WHO, Geneva, Switzerland (2012).
24. Smith SC Jr, Collins A, Ferrari R, et al. Our time: A call to save preventable death from cardiovascular disease (heart disease and stroke). *J Am Coll Cardiol.* 2012;60:2343–2348.
25. World Health Organization. Global Atlas CVD Prevention/Control. WHO, Geneva, Switzerland (2011).
26. Global Health Strategies Initiative. Shifting paradigm: How the BRICS are reshaping global health and development. 2012. http://www.ghsinitiatives.org/brics-report. Accessed June 02, 2016.
27. World Health Organization and World Economic Forum. From burden to "best buys": Reducing the economic impact of NCDs in low- and middle-income countries. WHO, Geneva, Switzerland (2011).
28. Nainggolan L. Doing nothing about CVD will cost $47 trillion. *Heartwire* (September 17, 2012) http://www.theheart.org/article/1447691.do. Accessed June 02, 2016.
29. Bloom DE, Cafiero ET, Jane-Llopis E, et al. The global economic burden of noncommunicable diseases. World Economic Forum, Geneva, Switzerland (2011).
30. World Heart Federation. Urbanization and cardiovascular disease: Raising heart-healthy children in today's cities. WHF, Geneva, Switzerland (2012).
31. Gaziano TA. Reducing the growing burden of cardiovascular disease in the developing world. *Health Aff (Millwood).* 2007;26(1):13–24.
32. Crimmins EM, Kim JK, Solé-Auró A. Gender differences in health: Results from SHARE, ELSA, and HRS. *Eur J Public Health.* 2011; 21(1):81–91.

CHAPTER 2

Pathophysiology

Garrett Ruth, MD, Garrett Brown, MD, Eileen Handberg, PhD, ARNP-BC, and R. David Anderson, MD, MS

PATHOPHYSIOLOGY

Coronary artery thrombosis is the final pathogenic mechanism in most cases of an acute coronary syndrome (ACS), as documented by angiographic and pathologic studies.[1,2] For example, coronary artery thrombi are found in 50% to 75% of cases of sudden cardiac death. Most commonly an ACS is accompanied by the formation of an intraluminal clot. Such clot formation is believed to result from the loss of a protective covering over an atherosclerotic plaque. In healthy arteries, the protective layer of endothelial cells separates the blood from potentially thrombogenic elements of the subintimal or the medial layer (**Figure 2.1**, left). In unhealthy arterial vessels, the development of atherosclerotic plaque may occur, which compromises the integrity of this protective layer of cells. The so-called cap on the surface of the plaque usually involves inflammatory cells. This cap may be thicker and more stable, or thinner and less stable, which is often called vulnerable plaque. An ACS usually begins when there is a compromise in the cap. These events are episodes called plaque rupture or erosion. This disruption in the atherosclerotic cap allows blood to come in contact with highly thrombogenic components of the plaque's necrotic core and initiates the process of luminal thrombosis.[3,4] Intraluminal thrombosis has also been observed after exposure of blood to calcified nodules. Where on the

Acute Coronary Syndrome: Urgent and Follow-up Care © 2017
Joseph S. Alpert, Lynne T. Braun, Barbara J. Fletcher, Gerald Fletcher, Editors-in-Chief,
Cardiotext Publishing, ISBN: 978-1-935395-94-2

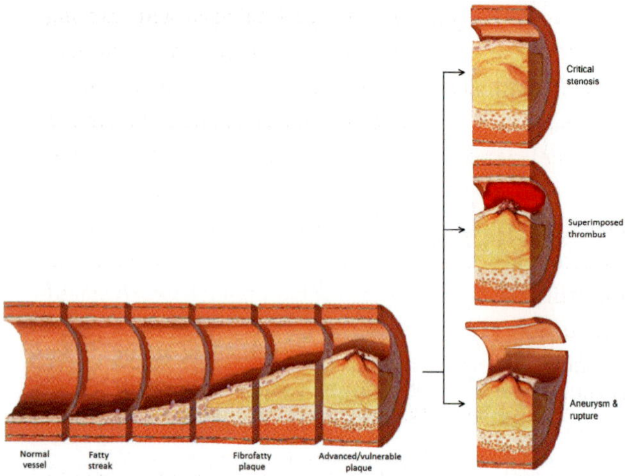

Figure 2.1

Progression of atherosclerotic disease leading to acute coronary syndrome. (*Source:* Wikipedia https://en.wikipedia.org/wiki/File:Atherosclerosis_disease_progression.png#filelinks, Licensed under the Creative Commons Attribution-ShareAlike 3.0 license http://creativecommons.org/licenses/by-sa/3.0/.)

spectrum of ACS a given patient resides ultimately depends on the degree of thrombosis that occurs.

Acute intraluminal thrombosis is characterized by aggregates of layered platelets and variable amounts of fibrin, red blood cells, and acute inflammatory cells. Insights into the mechanisms of coronary thrombosis have come from detailed analyses of plaque morphologies in cases of sudden death and acute myocardial infarction (AMI).[3,5–10]

Plaque rupture is the most common mechanism associated with acute coronary thrombosis. The morphology of plaque rupture shows an intraluminal thrombus overlying a thin disrupted fibrous cap covering an atherosclerotic plaque. The cap is infiltrated by macrophages and T-lymphocytes on an advanced lesion with a relatively large necrotic core.[3] The fibrous cap consists mainly of type I collagen with varying degrees of macrophages and lymphocytes, whereas the smooth muscle cells component within the cap is absent or sparse.

A breach in the fibrous cap allows circulating cellular and noncellular elements of blood to come in direct contact with the highly thrombogenic components of the necrotic core and is thought to be directly responsible for the actual development of the thrombus. Historically, the necrotic core was thought to be the main source of tissue factor; however, it is now believed that circulating monocytes, instead of macrophages alone, supply tissue factor that trigger and propagate the acute thrombi overlying unstable coronary atherosclerosis.[11] At the rupture site, the luminal thrombus often is platelet-rich thereby giving rise to a grossly white appearance (white thrombus), while at the proximal and distal ends near the sites of propagation it appears red (red thrombus) as it is composed of layers of fibrin and red blood cells.

Plaque erosion represents the second most prevalent underlying morphology of acute coronary thrombosis and is more common in women. In plaque erosion, the characteristics of the overlying thrombus differ significantly from those seen with in patients with plaque rupture. Autopsy studies of sudden death victims have shown that >85% of thrombi in erosions exhibited late stages of healing characterized by inflammatory cell lysis, invasion by smooth muscle cells and/or endothelial cells, or organized layers of smooth muscle cells and proteoglycans with varying degrees of platelet/fibrin layering, whereas in ruptures only one-half of thrombi show healing.[12]

Postmortem studies have shown that coronary thrombi superimposed on eroded plaques contain a higher density of myeloperoxidase-positive cells than thrombi superimposed on ruptured plaques.[13] Systemic myeloperoxidase levels are also elevated in patients with ACS presenting with eroded plaque compared with those presenting with rupture, suggesting that elevations in selective inflammatory biomarkers may reflect specific acute coronary events.[14]

An intense accumulation of extracellular matrix molecules such as hyaluronan and versican (proteoglycan) are observed at the sites of plaque erosion whereas there is relatively little accumulation of these factors at sites of plaque rupture.[15] It is hypothesized that a selective accumulation of hyaluronan in eroded plaques may promote the de-endothelialization and platelet aggregation. Hyaluronan can directly promote the polymerization of fibrin, which may facilitate smooth muscle cell migration and plaque progression.

The calcified nodule represents the least frequent underlying initiating pathology of luminal thrombus.[16] This term is reserved for fibrocalcific plaques with little or no underlying necrotic core associated with disruption of the luminal surface and thrombosis attributed to eruptive dense calcified nodules (**Figure 2.2**).

These occur in heavily calcified arteries and often show large plates of calcified matrix with surrounding areas of fibrosis, inflammation, and neovascularization. Although the precise nature of this lesion remains incompletely understood, fragmentation of the calcified plates may contribute to nodular calcification and sometimes bone formation can be observed with interspersed fibrin. The calcified nodule erodes into the lumen and the overlying collagen is thinned along with endothelial loss allowing the bare calcium to be in contact with the flowing blood and thrombus formation to occur. These lesions are generally more prevalent in older males with tortuous coronary arteries and chronic renal failure.

Additional information about the prevalence, distribution, and outcomes of patients with calcified nodules comes from PROSPECT study.[17] Three-vessel gray-scale and virtual histology intravascular ultrasound (IVUS) was performed in the proximal-mid-segments of all three coronary arteries in 697 patients with an ACS who underwent stenting. Investigators

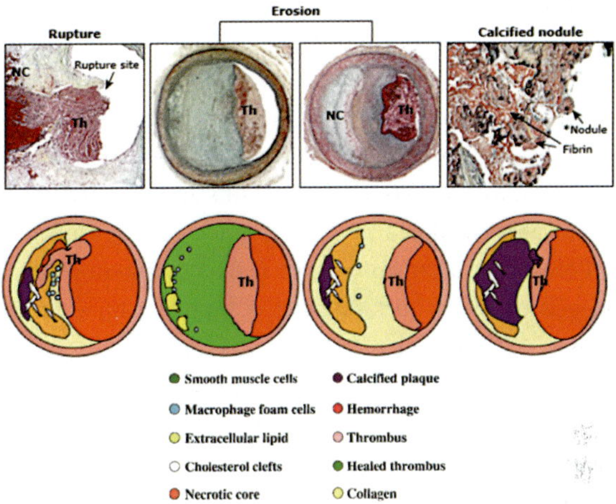

Figure 2.2

Differing plaques features leading to acute thrombosis. (*Source:* Virmani R, Kolodgie FD, Burke AP, et al. Lessons from sudden coronary death: A comprehensive morphological classification scheme for atherosclerotic lesions. *Arterioscler Thromb Vasc Biol.* 2000;20:1262–1275. Used with permission.)

found that calcified nodules were present in about 30% of patients. They appeared most commonly in the more proximal portions of the left coronary arteries but were present more diffusely in the right coronary arteries. Patients with calcified nodules were older, had more plaque volume and thicker caps, and fewer adverse events in 3 years of follow-up. Caution must be exercised, however, when interpreting these results, as most of the IVUS-detected calcified nodules in this study did not have significant thrombus. Many previously reported pathologic studies required the presence of luminal thrombus associated with calcified nodules to explain an ACS. The exact role of calcified nodules in the initiation of an ACS remains controversial, particularly with the absence of thrombus.[18]

Nonatherosclerotic ACS

Atherosclerotic disease underlies the majority of the clinical conditions in the spectrum of ACS, where some degree of coronary narrowing and plaque compromise can lead to decreased perfusion in myocardium. However, there are other conditions with different mechanisms and pathophysiology that can also result in an ACS.

Prinzmetal's variant angina is a presentation of an ACS that is associated with vasospasm of the coronary arteries. As opposed to atherosclerotic disease, many of these patients present with anginal type pain at rest rather than with exertion. This can lead to transient ST elevations leading to myocardial ischemia. The pathophysiology behind Prinzmetal's variant angina is not fully understood. It is suspected to be associated with alterations in vascular smooth muscle cells that become exposed to cell mediators such as catecholamines, thromboxane A2, serotonin, histamine, and endothelin, leading to coronary artery vasoconstriction.[19] Other mechanisms that have been proposed include generalized endothelial dysfunction that either impairs vasodilation due to decreased production and release of intrinsic nitric oxide, and/or disrupts phosphorylation of myosin light chains, an integral part of smooth muscle contraction.[20] Studies have also shown that the autonomic system plays a role in Prinzmetal's angina. Imbalances in the parasympathetic tone in comparison with the alpha-adrenergic receptors can lead to persistent vasospasm.[21]

Coronary artery dissection, also known as spontaneous coronary artery dissection (SCAD), is a rare but documented cause of ACS. This syndrome typically occurs in young females and occurs in the peripartum period. Uncommonly, it can occur in those with atherosclerotic disease. In the group associated with the peripartum period, dissection most commonly occurs 2 weeks following delivery.[22] The pathophysiology is not well studied but is presumed to be associated with variations in the levels of sex hormones. High levels of estrogen are hypothesized to alter the arterial wall composition, specifically hypertrophy of smooth muscle cells that loosen the intercellular matrix in the setting of increased acid mucopolysaccarides, leading to spontaneous dissections.[23] Also contributing to this is an elevation in baseline metabolic function including increased cardiac output, blood volume, and heart rate which add to the shearing forces on the coronary circulation leading to elevated wall stress.

Another population associated with SCAD is young women with nonobstructive atherosclerotic disease. In a study by Herin et al., 35 of 42 SCAD patients (nonpregnant) who had IVUS during cardiac catheterization were found to have atherosclerotic disease.[24] The mechanism of dissection does not seem to be related to hormonal changes but has been reasoned to be associated with increased density of the vasovasorum from atherosclerotic disease, leading to dissection of adventitia from the media and rupture of the intima.[25]

Coronary arterial inflammation in relation to various systemic disease states, including systemic lupus erythematosus, rheumatoid arthritis, and individual vasculitides, can lead to coronary artery disease (CAD) and ACS. Both the epicardial arteries and the microvascular coronary arteries can be affected depending on the disease state. In coronary vasculitis the composition of the inflammatory cells includes B cells, in contrast to atherosclerotic disease which involves mostly mononuclear cells. The distribution of inflammation can also be used to help distinguish the different diseases. Typically in vasculitis the entire arterial wall possesses inflammatory markers with prominence in the adventitia. Inflammation in atherosclerotic disease is mostly confined to the intima. However, in advanced atherosclerotic disease the adventitia can develop some degree of inflammation as well.[26]

The most well recognized form of coronary vasculitis occurs in Kawasaki disease which most commonly affects the coronary circulation leading to a high incidence of acquired heart disease in the pediatric population. Coronary aneurysms tend to develop which is believed to be due to fibrocellular intimal proliferation leading to swelling and filling of the aneurysmal sac.[27]

Another increasingly recognized cause of ACS is **microvascular dysfunction (MVD)** or **"cardiac syndrome X."** Although sometimes associated with atherosclerosis, patients with MVD present with anginal symptoms in the absence of any cardiac or systemic disease. Diagnostic testing including ECGs and stress testing show no evidence indicative of myocardial ischemia. It has been suggested that MVD occurs more commonly in the female population.[28] However, some data do show a more even distribution between males and females.[29] Studies have suggested the pathophysiology of MVD is multifactorial, owing to both structural and functional abnormalities. Structural changes include smooth muscle hypertrophy of the microvasculature resulting in decreased coronary blood flow.[30] Functionally, it has been proposed that reduced nitric oxide-releasing mechanisms lead to dysfunction in the vasodilation of the dependent endothelium. This has been demonstrated by invasive angiography with reduced coronary blood flow in response to acetylcholine or adenosine.[31] In a study by Desideri et al., the metabolics of nitric oxide did not seem to be affected despite acetylcholine administration which indicated additional pathways may play a role in MVD.[32]

Elevated biomarkers are typically associated with acute or subacute myocardial damage. Clinical scenarios other than acute thrombotic occlusion can also lead to release of cardiac enzymes. One scenario is known as **demand ischemia** which may lead to a **type 2 myocardial infarction (MI)**. By definition, the 2012 Joint ESC universal definition of type 2 MI is when the event is secondary to ischemia due to either an increased oxygen demand or decreased supply in the absence of an acute primary coronary thrombotic event.[33] Oxygen demand is elevated in many common clinical settings such as sepsis, septic shock, and systemic inflammatory response syndrome.[34] Tachyarrhythmias can also lead to transient elevations in cardiac enzymes due to alterations in cardiac output and oxygen consumption.[35]

Finally, an ACS can less commonly be caused by **nonatherosclerotic coronary thrombosis** in the setting of **hypercoagulability** or other chronic disease states. This group includes patients with embolic phenomena that can occur in the setting of atrial tachyarrhythmias. Patients with atrial fibrillation or flutter who are at increased risk of thromboembolism can present with an MI as their first manifestation of left atrial appendage. Clinical conditions such as Protein C/S deficiency, Factor V Leiden, oral contraceptive use, and smoking have been documented to have an increased risk of AMI with normal coronary angiograms.[36] Factor V Leiden is a common risk factor for venous thromboembolism which can occur in up to 10% of this population and more than half of patients with hypercoagulable states.[36] One particular population study estimated that 36% of patients with AMI with normal coronary angiograms possess at least one inheritable factor of thrombophilia compared to 6% of healthy controls.[37] In women, estrogens have been postulated to have a prothrombotic effect leading to increased binding from fibrinogen in comparison to men.[38] A study of women who presented with AMI in the setting of normal angiography showed a higher prevalence in those pregnant or on exogenous estrogen (34%) versus a healthy control group (14%).[39] Tobacco use is highly associated with atherosclerotic disease. However, in those with normal coronary arteries who smoke it has been suggested that due to direct tPA inhibitory activity[40] along with nitric oxide suppression[41] can lead to acute coronary thrombosis.

REFERENCES

1. DeWood MA, Spores J, Notske R, et al. Prevalence of total coronary occlusion during the early hours of transmural myocardial infarction. *N Engl J Med.* 1980;303(16):897–902.

2. Falk E. Unstable angina with fatal outcome: Dynamic coronary thrombosis leading to infarction and/or sudden death. Autopsy evidence of recurrent mural thrombosis with peripheral embolization culminating in total vascular occlusion. *Circulation.* 1985;71:699–708.
3. Virmani R, Kolodgie FD, Burke AP, et al. Lessons from sudden coronary death: A comprehensive morphological classification scheme for atherosclerotic lesions. *Arterioscler Thromb Vasc Biol.* 2000;20:1262–1275.
4. Burke AP, Farb A, Malcom GT, et al. Plaque rupture and sudden death related to exertion in men with coronary artery disease. *JAMA.* 1999;281:921–926.
5. Davies MJ, Thomas A. Thrombosis and acute coronary-artery lesions in sudden cardiac ischemic death. *N Engl J Med.* 1984;310:1137–1140.
6. el Fawal MA, Berg GA, Wheatley DJ, et al. Sudden coronary death in Glasgow: Nature and frequency of acute coronary lesions. *Br Heart J.* 1987;57:329–335.
7. Davies MJ, Bland JM, Hangartner JR, et al. Factors influencing the presence or absence of acute coronary artery thrombi in sudden ischaemic death. *Eur Heart J.* 1989;10:203–208.
8. Burke AP, Farb A, Malcom GT, et al. Coronary risk factors and plaque morphology in men with coronary disease who died suddenly. *N Engl J Med.* 1997;336:1276–1282.
9. Burke AP, Farb A, Malcom GT, et al. Effect of risk factors on the mechanism of acute thrombosis and sudden coronary death in women. *Circulation.* 1998;97:2110–2116.
10. Arbustini E, Dal Bello B, Morbini P, et al. Plaque erosion is a major substrate for coronary thrombosis in acute myocardial infarction. *Heart.* 1999;82:269–272.
11. Nemerson Y. A simple experiment and a weakening paradigm: The contribution of blood to propensity for thrombus formation. *Arterioscler Thromb Vasc Biol.* 2002;22:1369.
12. Kramer MC, Rittersma SZ, de Winter RJ, et al. Relationship of thrombus healing to underlying plaque morphology in sudden coronary death. *J Am Coll Cardiol.* 2010;55:122.
13. Ferrante G, Nakano M, Prati F, et al. High levels of systemic myeloperoxidase are associated with coronary plaque erosion in patients with acute coronary syndromes: A clinicopathological study. *Circulation.* 2010;122:2505.
14. Kolodgie FD, Burke AP, Farb A, et al. Differential accumulation of proteoglycans and hyaluronan in culprit lesions: Insights into plaque erosion. *Arterioscler Thromb Vasc Biol.* 2002;22:1642.
15. Xu Y, Mintz GS, Tam A, et al. Prevalence, distribution, predictors, and outcomes of patients with calcified nodules in native coronary arteries: A 3-vessel intravascular ultrasound analysis from Providing

Regional Observations to Study Predictors of Events in the Coronary Tree (PROSPECT). *Circulation.* 2012;126:537.

16. Ambrose JA, Tannenbaum MA, Alexopoulos D, et al. Angiographic progression of coronary artery disease and the development of myocardial infarction. *J Am Coll Cardiol.* 1988;12:56.
17. Glaser R, Selzer F, Faxon DP, et al. Clinical progression of incidental, asymptomatic lesions discovered during culprit vessel coronary intervention. *Circulation.* 2005;111:143.
18. Farb A, Burke AP, Tang AL, et al. Coronary plaque erosion without rupture into a lipid core. A frequent cause of coronary thrombosis in sudden coronary death. *Circulation.* 1996;93:1354.
19. Willerson JT, Hillis LD, Winniford M, et al. Speculation regarding mechanisms responsible for acute ischemic heart disease syndromes. *J Am Coll Cardiol.* 1986;8:245–250.
20. Kugiyama K, Yasue H, Okumura K, et al. Nitric oxide activity is deficient in spasm arteries of patients with coronary spastic angina. *Circulation.* 1996;94:266–271.
21. Yasue H, Horio Y, Nakamura N, et al. Induction of coronary artery spasm by acetylcholine in patients with variant angina: Possible role of the parasympathetic nervous system in the pathogenesis of coronary artery spasm. *Circulation.* 1986;74:955–963.
22. Koul AK, Hollander G, Moskovits N, et al. Coronary artery dissection during pregnancy and the postpartum period: Two case reports and review of literature. *Catheter Cardiovasc Interv.* 2001 Jan;52(1):88–94.
23. Asuncion CM, Hyun J. Dissecting intramural hematoma of the coronary artery in pregnancy and the puerperium. *Obstet Gynecol.* 1972 Aug;40(2):202–210.
24. Hering D, Piper C, Hohmann C, et al. Prospective study of the incidence, pathogenesis and therapy of spontaneous, by coronary angiography diagnosed coronary artery dissection. *Z Kardiol.* 1998 Dec; 87(12):961–970.
25. Cheung S, Mithani V, Watson RM. Healing of spontaneous coronary dissection in the context of glycoprotein IIB/IIIA inhibitor therapy: A case report. *Catheter Cardiovasc Interv.* 2000 Sep;51(1): 95–100.
26. van der Wal AC, Becker AE. Atherosclerotic plaque rupture—Pathologic basis of plaque stability and instability. *Cardiovasc Res.* 1999 Feb;41(2):334–344.
27. Kuijpers TW, Biezeveld M, Achterhuis A, et al. Longstanding obliterative panarteritis in Kawasaki disease: Lack of cyclosporin A effect. *Pediatrics.* 2003 Oct;112(4):986–992.
28. Zipes DP, Libby P, Bonow RO, et al. *Braunwald's Heart Disease: A Textbook of Cardiovascular Medicine.* 8 ed. Philadelphia, PA: Saunders-Elsevier. 2008.

29. Kaski JC. Cardiac syndrome X in women: The role of oestrogen deficiency. *Heart.* 2006 May;92(Suppl 3):iii5–iii9.
30. Opherk D, Zebe H, Weihe E, et al. Reduced coronary dilator capacity and ultrastructural changes of the myocardium in patients with angina pectoris but normal coronary arteriograms. *Circulation.* 1981;63:817–825.
31. Motz W, Vogt M, Rabenau O, et al. Evidence of endothelial dysfunction in coronary resistance vessels in patients with angina pectoris and and normal coronary angiograms. *Am J Cardiol.* 1991;68:996–1003.
32. Desideri G, Gaspardone A, Gentile M, et al. Endothelial activation in patients with cardiac syndrome X. *Circulation.* 2000;102:2359–2364.
33. Thygesen K, Alpert JS, Jaffe AS, et al. Third universal definition of myocardial infarction. Joint ESC/ACCF/AHA/WHF Task Force for the Universal Definition of Myocardial Infarction. *Circulation.* 2012;126(16):2020.
34. Ammann P, Maggiorini M, Bertel O, et al. Troponin as a risk factor for mortality in critically ill patients without acute coronary syndromes. *J Am Coll Cardiol.* 2003;41(11):2004.
35. Zellweger MJ, Schaer BA, Cron TA, et al. Elevated troponin levels in absence of coronary artery disease after supraventricular tachycardia. *Swiss Med Wkly.* 2003;133(31–32):439.
36. DeLoughery TG. Coagulation abnormalities and cardiovascular disease. *Curr Opin Lipidol.* 1999;10:443–448.
37. Lande G, Dantec V, Trossaert M, et al. Do inherited prothrombotic factors have a role in myocardial infarction with normal coronary arteriogram? *J Intern Med.* 1998;244:543–544.
38. Faraday N, Goldschmidt-Clermont PJ, Bray PF. Gender differences in platelet GPIIb-IIIa activation. *Thromb Haemost.* 1997;77:748–754.
39. Raymond R, Lynch J, Underwood D, et al. Myocardial infarction and normal coronary arteriography: A 10 year clinical and risk analysis of 74 patients. *J Am Coll Cardiol.* 1988;11:471–477.
40. Hamsten A, Wiman B, de Faire U, et al. Increased plasma levels of a rapid inhibitor of tissue plasminogen activator in young survivors of myocardial infarction. *N Engl J Med.* 1985;313:1557–1563.
41. Ichiki K, Ikeda H, Haramaki N, et al. Longterm smoking impairs platelet-derived nitric oxide release. *Circulation.* 1996;94:3109–3114.

CHAPTER 3

Outcomes

Garrett Ruth, MD, and R. David Anderson, MD, MS

Myocardial infarction (MI) as discussed in previous chapters carries a high risk of complications and death upon initial presentation. Patients who survive their first heart attack are subsequently at increased risk of morbidity and mortality. Although the overall prognosis can be influenced by many factors, it has been estimated that the in-hospital or 30-day mortality is around 2% to 3% when ST-segment elevation MI (STEMI), non-STEMI (NSTEMI), and unstable angina (UA) are included together.[1] This has notably decreased over the past 20 years with the advent of management of acute coronary syndrome (ACS) including antiplatelet agents, beta blockers, statins, and percutaneous coronary intervention (PCI).[2]

SHORT-TERM OUTCOMES

For STEMI patients, the 30-day mortality rate has ranged from 2% to 10% in various population studies.[3,4] Outcomes can be further divided into three treatment groups: 1) medical therapy, 2) fibrinolytic therapy, or 3) PCI. Medical therapy alone led to mortality rates as high as 13% in contrast to fibrinolytic therapy with mortality rates of about 6% to 7%.[5] The gold standard treatment with cardiac catheterization and PCI reduced mortality to as low as 3% to 5%.[6,7] It is important to note that these trials included door-to-balloon times of less than 2 hours starting from the onset of chest pain. A 2012 study (6000 patients presenting with an STEMI over a span of 10 years) demonstrated significant improvements in mortality

Acute Coronary Syndrome: Urgent and Follow-up Care © 2017
Joseph S. Alpert, Lynne T. Braun, Barbara J. Fletcher, Gerald Fletcher, Editors-in-Chief,
Cardiotext Publishing, ISBN: 978-1-935395-94-2

since the early 1990s.[8] Overall since 1995, 30-day mortality, which was greater than 13%, has steadily declined to 4% independent of the type of treatment. Other notable findings are increased recognition of ACS in younger women (<60 years of age), changes in population characteristics of STEMIs, and increased use and compliance of ACS treatment.[8]

In the case of NSTEMI patients, 30-day mortality rates are lower when compared with those presenting with an STEMI. Specifically, for NSTEMI, the incidence of in-hospital morality was around 2% to 3% in large nonrandomized studies.[9] In the Global Registry of Acute Coronary Events (GRACE) registry including over 16,000 patients from various countries enrolled between 2001 and 2007, those presenting with an NSTEMI had an overall in-hospital mortality rate of 3.3%.[10]

LONG-TERM OUTCOMES

As stated previously, patients who present with NSTEMI have been shown to have a more favorable 30-day mortality rate. However, when considering longer outcomes, multiple studies have revealed conflicting data.

In the Global Use of Strategies to Open Occluded Coronary Arteries in Acute Coronary Syndromes (GUSTO-IIb), performed in the 1990s, the 1-year mortality rates of NSTEMI versus STEMI were comparable.[11] NSTEMI had an 8.8% 1-year mortality rate, while the STEMI rate was 9.6%.[11] In contrast to the GUSTO study, the OPERA registry studied 2000 patients who presented with acute MI (AMI) and underwent percutaneous intervention or fibrinolytic therapy for ACS treatment. The data showed that the mortality at 1-year follow up was higher in NSTEMI at 8.2%, versus 5% in patients who met STEMI criteria.[12]

Another two studies performed at similar times in the early to middle 2000s continued to suggest that NSTEMI leads to poorer long-term outcomes. In a French data set, 1600 patients with NSTEMI who underwent cardiac catheterization revealed a 3-year mortality rate as high as 20%, with half of the deaths attributed to a cardiac etiology.[13] In the HORIZONS-AMI trial, STEMI patients who underwent PCI had a comparatively lower 3-year mortality rate of only 6% to 7%.[14] It has been hypothesized that the increased mortality seen in NSTEMI patients is due in part to advanced stage multivessel disease leading to frequent recurrent ischemia and recurrent MI.[11]

One single-center study in a large population studied individual classification of ACS including UA, minor myocardial damage (MMD, defined at the time as elevated creatine kinase MB isoenzyme with normal total creatine kinase), NSTEMI, and STEMI to assess long-term outcome and mortality. Of 760 patients identified and distributed by clinical presentation, 22% presented with UA, 35% had MMD, 26% had NSTEMI, and 17% presented with STEMI. The data showed that MMD/NSTEMI was associated with poorer 10-year survival following hospitalization (**Figures 3.1** and **3.2**).[15]

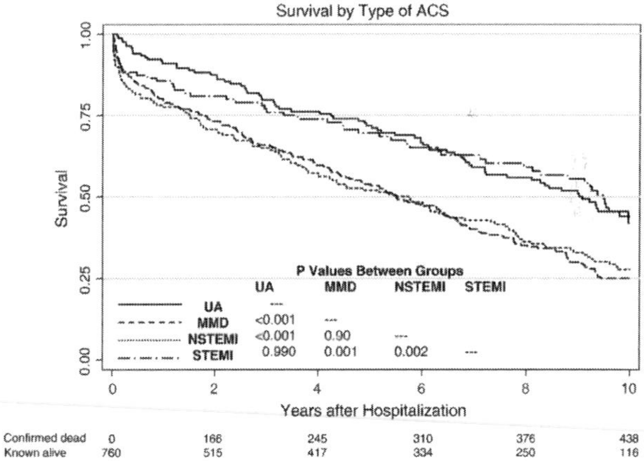

Figure 3.1

Unadjusted 10-year Kaplan-Meier survival curves.

(*Source:* Allen LA, O'Donnell CJ, Camargo CA, Jr., et al. Comparison of long-term mortality across the spectrum of acute coronary syndromes. *Am Heart J.* 2006 May;151(5):1065–1071. Used with permission.)

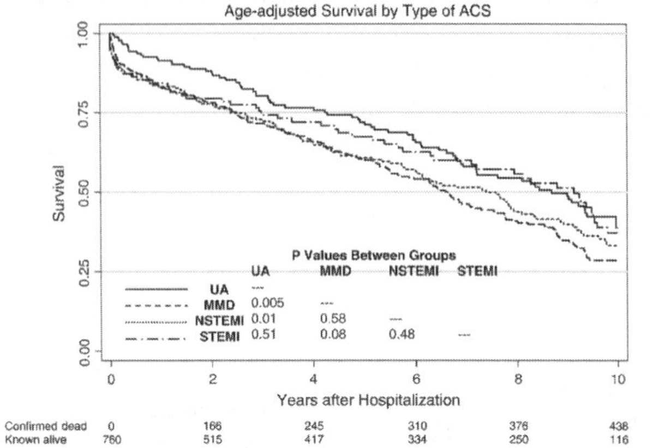

Age-adjusted survival curves up to 10 years from index hospitalization, stratified by type of ACS presentation.

Figure 3.2

Age-adjusted 10-year Kaplan–Meier survival curves.

(*Source:* Allen LA, O'Donnell CJ, Camargo CA, Jr., et al. Comparison of long-term mortality across the spectrum of acute coronary syndromes. *Am Heart J.* 2006 May;151(5):1065–1071. Used with permission.)

With NSTEMI/MMD it was hypothesized that one of the contributing factors leading to increased long-term mortality was the higher burden of comorbidities rather than the STEMI cohorts who predominantly presented with initial first-time MI.[15]

A more recent study similarly comparing the different clinical presentations of ACS published in 2009 from the Netherlands specifically looked at the mortality after PCI. Between 1997 and 2005, over 10,000 patients in this cohort underwent PCI (28% STEMI, 32% UA/NSTEMI, and 40% stable angina).[16] The authors revealed that the mortality rates at 6 years for STEMI patients was 18.9% versus 16.2% in those with UA/NSTEMI and 11.7% with stable angina.[16] A significant finding was that patients with STEMI demonstrated a greater 6-month mortality than UA/STEMI (relative risk [RR] 3.09,

95% confidence interval [CI] 2.46–3.98) and stable angina (RR 5.82, 95% CI 4.45–7.65).[16] However, compared with the previous trial, it was noted that after 6 months to 6 years the greatest incidence of mortality were in those patients with UA/NSTEMI (UA/NSTEMI vs. stable angina: RR 1.33, 95% CI 1.1–1.58; STEMI vs. UA/NSTEMI: RR 0.80, 95% CI 0.65–0.99).[16] **Figures 3.3–3.5** demonstrate the different clinical presentations and their survival following cardiac catheterization.

FACTORS AFFECTING OUTCOMES

Risk stratification prior to MI includes identifying those patients at higher risk for cardiac disease. It is also important

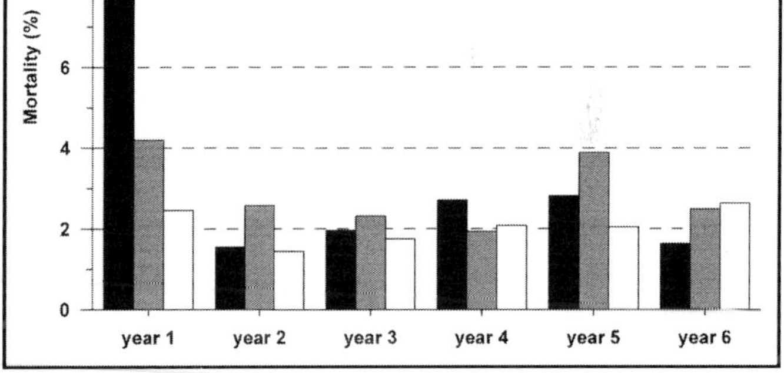

Figure 3.3

Bar graph of mortality rates for STEMI, UA/NSTEMI, and stable angina.

Hirsch A, Verouden NJ, Koch KT, et al. Comparison of long-term mortality after percutaneous coronary intervention in patients treated for acute ST-elevation myocardial infarction versus those with unstable and stable angina pectoris. (*Source: Am J Cardiol.* 2009 Aug;104(3):333–337. Used with permission.)

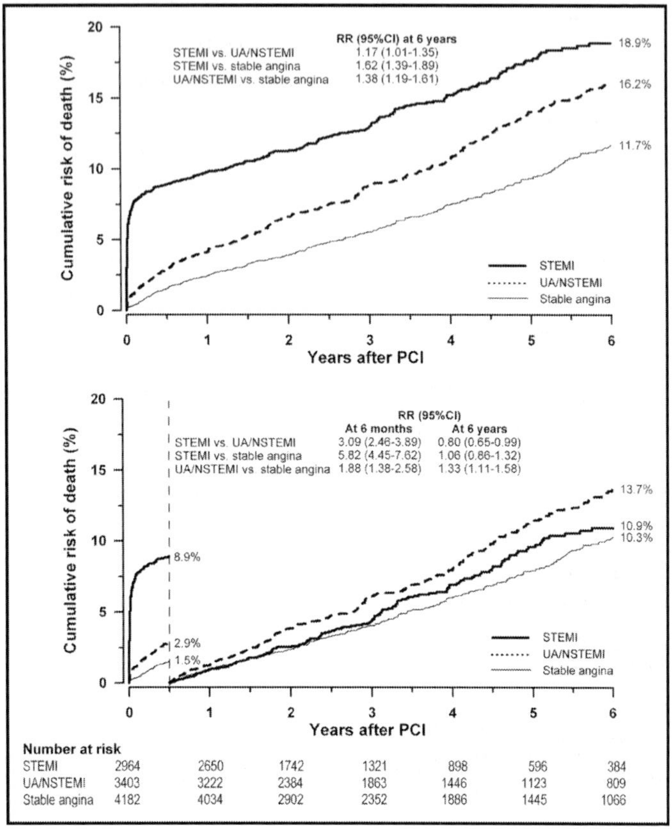

Figure 3.4

Unadjusted survival rates.

Hirsch A, Verouden NJ, Koch KT, et al. Comparison of long-term mortality after percutaneous coronary intervention in patients treated for acute ST-elevation myocardial infarction versus those with unstable and stable angina pectoris. (*Source: Am J Cardiol.* 2009 Aug;104(3):333–337. Used with permission.)

after a patient suffers their first MI to consider these risk factors as they play a significant role in both short- and long-term outcomes.

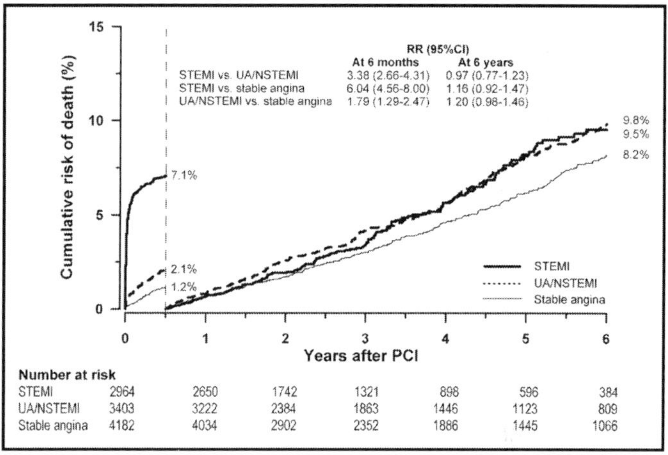

Figure 3.5

Adjusted survival rates.

Hirsch A, Verouden NJ, Koch KT, et al. Comparison of long-term mortality after percutaneous coronary intervention in patients treated for acute ST-elevation myocardial infarction versus those with unstable and stable angina pectoris. (*Source: Am J Cardiol.* 2009 Aug;104(3):333–337. Used with permission.)

Peripheral arterial disease or symptoms of recurrent intermittent claudication have been associated with poorer outcomes. In one study, patients who reported claudication-type symptoms with recent MI were found to have 19.2% mortality versus those without symptoms at 3.6%.[17] This is likely related to the fact that having vascular disease in at least two territories is a marker of more severe comorbidities.

Chronic kidney disease has been studied extensively in the setting of MI. In a review of patients hospitalized with AMI, 1-year mortality was directly related to an increase in serum creatinine. For those patients with a creatinine of ≤1.5 mg/dL mortality was significantly lower than that seen in patients with a serum creatinine >2.5.[18] In the VALIANT trial, 14,000 patients had estimated glomerular filtration rates compared after AMI, and there was a direct correlation between declining renal function and worsening outcomes.[19]

Post-MI **atrial fibrillation** has also been shown to have an impact on outcome. Atrial fibrillation was recorded in a large population study (GISSI-3) and occurred at a rate of 6.7% to 7.6% after MI.[20] In patients who developed atrial fibrillation, the exact onset of the dysrhythmia was related proportionally to an increase in mortality. Those who developed atrial fibrillation within the first few days after AMI were found to have a hazard ratio of 1.63 (95% CI: 1.37–1.93), while developing this dysrhythmia after 1 month conveyed a hazard ratio of 2.58 (95% CI: 2.21–3.00).[21]

Recurrent ischemia is also a poor prognostic sign after AMI. This includes both symptoms of angina and silent markers of ischemia. Typically, those patients with recurring ischemia are at higher risk for reinfarction. Using the GUSTO-IIb trial, 4125 patients with STEMI were divided into three groups: 1) patients without recurrent ischemia, 2) recurrent ischemia responding to medial therapy, and 3) refractory ischemia. Respectively, the mortality rates were 2.7%, 11%, and 28% at 30 days, and there was a tendency to further increase at 6 months and 1 year.[11]

COMPLICATIONS OF ACUTE MYOCARDIAL INFARCTION

Following MI, patients are at increased risk of complications ranging from minor pain to life-threatening conditions. These conditions encompass different processes related to mechanical dysfunction, immunologic response, infection, or generalized inflammation. Typically, the symptoms associated with various complications following AMI can be used in conjunction with the patient's clinical presentation and can help one establish a diagnosis.

A common diagnosis following MI is **pericarditis**. Pericarditis post-AMI involves a noninfectious inflammatory response of the pericardium to the recent myocardial injury and can be associated with audible friction rub on auscultation. In one study, pericarditis occurred in 5% of patients who received fibrinolytic therapy during AMI compared with 12% to 20% who received medical therapy alone.[22,23] The clinical significance of a friction rub when discovered 2 to 3 days post-MI has been observed to indicate a higher incidence of 1-year mortality as it has been associated with larger areas of ischemia, systolic dysfunction, and higher troponin levels.[24] One prospective study with 743 patients presenting with STEMI showed a 4.2% incidence of diagnosed pericarditis.[25] Each patient underwent percutaneous intervention. It was recognized in this study that the prevalence of pericarditis was directly related to the time of presentation and interval to catheterization. Pericarditis was observed in 1.7% of patients in <3 hours, 5.4% in 3–6 hours, and 13.6% in >3 hours.[25] Early revascularization has been previously shown to have a clear mortality benefit but may also reduce the incidence of post-MI pericarditis.

Another potential complication of MI related to pericarditis is **pericardial effusion.** Pericardial effusions may be seen in up to one-third of patients presenting with STEMI. In a review of 330 patients from Osaka, Japan who presented with a STEMI, 83 patients (25%) had echocardiographic evidence of pericardial effusion post-MI.[26] Many of these effusions were mild and did not contribute to a significant increase in morbidity or mortality. However, in one retrospective study, 228 patients who were found to have more severe, moderate to large effusions (>10 mm) experienced a higher 30-day mortality (10% vs. 6%) compared with those with lower volume effusions.[27]

Cardiac tamponade occurs when a pericardial effusion, whether by its volume or the rapidity of accumulation, exceeds the heart's ability to compensate for it which leads to hemodynamic compromise. This serious and life-threatening complication occurs rarely but must be recognized promptly for appropriate management. In a large study conducted by the Duke Clinical Research Institute in 2006, over 100,000 patients who presented with AMI (specifically STEMI) were included. The authors found that only 0.85% (865) of AMI patients developed clinically significant cardiac tamponade.[28] Of those 865 patients, the population was predominantly older (median age 71.9 years), female (54%), associated more with anterior MI (61.9%), and had a longer time to reperfusion.[28] It is important to note that all of the patients analyzed were treated with fibrinolytic reperfusion strategies. In patients who undergo PCI, other studies have shown a much lower incidence of tamponade. In a study from William Beaumont Hospital in Royal Oak, Michigan among 25,000 patients who had PCI for AMI, only 31 patients (0.12%) were found to have clinically significant cardiac tamponade.[29] Another trial with 7,000 patients who had PCI reported an incidence of 0.2%, still a substantial decrease from the large Duke clinical database treated with fibrinolytic therapy.[30] This has been hypothesized to be due to the lessened amount of myocardial necrosis with successful intervention, suggesting that time to reperfusion also plays a key role in complications such as tamponade.[28] It is probable that the rate of true spontaneous tamponade may actually be lower, as the above numbers likely included events related to cardiac catheterization procedures.

Postcardiac injury syndrome, more commonly known as **Dressler's syndrome**, is a condition seen in patients who have an AMI, recover, and then experience symptoms similar to those of pericarditis within months of the initial insult. This syndrome has occurred less frequently since the advent of PCI and fibrinolytic reperfusion strategies. Initially described by Dressler in 1959, 44 case reports were studied and described the complication as "idiopathic, recurrent, benign pericarditis."[31]

In a more recent but limited study from Tel Aviv University in Israel, 201 patients were followed for 3 months after AMI. Each patient underwent fibrinolytic therapy followed by heparin infusion for treatment of AMI. Only one patient of the group was clinically diagnosed with Dressler's syndrome, and this patient did not have evidence of early reperfusion.[32] The pathogenesis has been hypothesized to reflect an immunologic response to previously injured myocardium releasing cardiac antigens leading to antibody formation. Antibodies then begin to deposit in affected areas such as the pericardium and pleura, which over time leads to an inflammatory response and symptoms.[33]

Left-ventricular free wall rupture rarely occurs in patients who suffer a devastating STEMI with widespread necrosis. One study observed 849 patients who presented with STEMI and rupture occurred in only 14 cases (1.7%).[34] However, the cohort demonstrated that three characteristics put specific patients at higher risk (9.2 times more likely) of free wall rupture. These included no prior history of MI, ST segment elevation with evidence of Q-wave transition indicating late stage infarction, and high levels of creatine kinase MB (>150 IU/L).[34] When encompassing all AMI, free wall rupture is rare. In a single-center study from Spain, over 6678 patients who presented with STEMI were analyzed from the years 1977 to 2006, divided into different 5-year periods. The overall free wall rupture rate was 4%, but this rate declined over advancing years as fibrinolytics and PCI strategies became more commonly used, suggesting that the use of reperfusion therapy led to smaller infarcts and lower rates of free wall rupture.[35] Over 50% of free wall ruptures occur within the first 5 days following AMI, while 90% occur in the first 2 weeks.[36] There tends to be a bimodal morphologic distribution between early versus late-stage rupture, as studied in a population in Osaka, Japan, in which 27 of 1450 patients had clinical free wall rupture following STEMI. On pathological examination the early ruptures were characteristically "a slit like tear in the affected myocardium, with preference for anterior MI sites." The late-stage ruptures consisted of infarct expansion with no specific site in patients who had experienced failed reperfusion.[36]

Another serious mechanical complication of MI is the occurrence of **ventricular septal rupture (VSR)** or a **ventricular septal defect (VSD)**. The pathogenesis of septal defect formation is related to coagulation necrosis of the injured or scarred myocardium after infarction, with neutrophilic inflammation leading to thinning and destruction of the ventricular wall.[37] In various population studies, VSR has been demonstrated to occur at around half the rate of those with free wall ruptures. In the previously mentioned Spanish study in 6678 patients presenting with an STEMI, only 145 suffered VSR.[35] Again, as the incidence of free wall rupture declined with the advent of reperfusion therapy, the incidence of VSR also decreased.[35] In the GUSTO-I trial, VSD complicated an AMI in only 84 (0.2%) of 41,021 patients, a lower incidence than among patients without successful reperfusion.[38] Risk factors for VSR/VSD include advanced age, hypertension, anterior MI, unsuccessful or no reperfusion therapy, and female gender.[37] Specifically, the incidence has been observed to be increased in patients with single-vessel left anterior descending (LAD) artery disease, extensive myocardial injury, and ischemia with poor collateralization.[39] The occurrence is also increased in diffuse multivessel disease, but not to the extent of that in single-vessel disease.[40] This is likely due to increased collateral blood flow in the setting of chronic obstruction[40] as well as the LAD artery supplying the majority of the septal vasculature. In some instances, the LAD extends beyond the apex of the heart to supply distal branches of the inferior wall, contributing an even larger portion of circulation to the septum. In one study, the incidence of VSR was recorded and compared with ECG findings consistent with abnormal Q-wave presence in inferior versus a control group of anterior MI without inferior ECG changes.[41] The results showed that inferior Q waves (hypothesizing a "wrap around" left anterior descending artery providing a significant portion of septal blood flow) appeared in 44.4% of patients with VSR and in only 4.0% of patients without VSR.[41] It is important to recognize symptoms and complications of VSR as patients frequently become unstable and require urgent surgical intervention. In those 84 patients in the GUSTO-I trial that suffered VSR, surgical repair was performed in 40% within 3.5 days of symptom onset, and survival was significantly improved in those who underwent surgical management versus those who did not, respectively, at both 30 days (53% vs. 6% survival) and 1 year (47% vs. 3%).[38]

Ischemic mitral regurgitation following AMI, both acute and chronic, can be caused by various etiologies including papillary muscle dysfunction, left-ventricular dilation, or chordae tendineae rupture. Acute mitral regurgitation can be common in post-MI patients, and the degree of dysfunction has an impact on overall mortality. In the SHOCK trial, 169 patients were assessed by echocardiography following MI, and moderate to severe mitral regurgitation was detected in 39%.[42] More importantly, this finding correlated with a poorer survival rate at 1-year follow-up compared with those with mild to no mitral regurgitation (31% vs. 58%).[42] Despite this, many patients who are found to have mitral regurgitation post-MI can have functional recovery of the left ventricle (LV) following revascularization and appropriate medical therapy. Alternatively, patients can have permanently fixed mitral dysfunction and require mitral valve repair or replacement. In a study performed by the American Heart Association, 2757 patients who underwent catheterization between 1986 and 2001 who had moderate mitral regurgitation (by echocardiography) were stratified into four treatment groups: 1) medical treatment alone, 2) PCI, 3) coronary artery bypass surgery, and 4) coronary artery bypass surgery with mitral valve surgery. In the PCI group there was a 31% risk reduction (hazard ratio = 0.69, $p = 0.0001$), versus bypass surgery having a 42% risk reduction (hazard ratio 0.58, $p = 0.0001$), and bypass with mitral valve surgery also resulting in a 42% risk reduction (hazard ratio 0.58, $p = 0.0001$).[43]

With papillary muscle rupture, mitral regurgitation becomes a life-threatening emergency following AMI. Typically this complication occurs within a week of the initial insult. An analysis of 17 patients who were diagnosed with papillary muscle rupture had a mean presentation of 6 days after MI.[44] In many cases the posteromedial papillary muscle is frequently involved due to the lack of dual blood supply that the anterolateral papillary muscle has, from both LAD and left circumflex coronary arteries.[45] As with the previous mechanical complications, papillary rupture requires rapid diagnosis followed by emergent surgery to reduce risk of death.

Patient outcomes following an ACS vary depending on comorbidities, initial clinical presentation, patient characteristics, and the use and success of treatment strategies. Survival following an ACS presentation has significantly improved over the past several decades with new reperfusions strategies and the widespread application of evidence-based medical management. Despite this, ACS patients must continue to be managed after the acute period with a multidisciplinary team in an effort to reduce risks and appropriately manage complications that may arise. Although the prevalence of ACS and its complications have been shown to be decreasing over time, the burden of disease with an overall increasing population will continue to play a significant role in the future of health care and the way these conditions are managed.

REFERENCES

1. Roe MT, Messenger JC, Weintraub WS, et al. Treatments, trends, and outcomes of acute myocardial infarction and percutaneous coronary intervention. *J Am Coll Cardiol.* 2010;56:254–263.
2. Rogers WJ, Frederick PD, Stoehr E, et al. Trends in presenting characteristics and hospital mortality among patients with ST

elevation and non-ST elevation myocardial infarction in the National Registry of Myocardial Infarction from 1990 to 2006. *Am Heart J.* 2008;156:1026–1034.

3. Rosamond WD, Chambless LE, Heiss G, et al. Twenty-two-year trends in incidence of myocardial infarction, coronary heart disease mortality, and case fatality in 4 U.S. communities, 1987–2008. *Circulation.* 2012;125:1848–1857.
4. Jernberg T, Johanson P, Held C, et al. Association between adoption of evidence-based treatment and survival for patients with ST-elevation myocardial infarction. *JAMA.* 2011;305:1677–1684.
5. Assessment of the Safety and Efficacy of a New Thrombolytic (ASSENT-2) Investigators, Van De Werf F, Adgey J, Ardissino D. Single-bolus tenecteplase compared with front-loaded alteplase in acute myocardial infarction: The ASSENT-2 double-blind randomised trial. *Lancet.* 1999;354:716–722.
6. Tobbia P, Brodie BR, Witzenbichler B, et al. Adverse event rates following primary PCI for STEMI at U.S. and non-U.S. hospitals: Three-year analysis from the HORIZONS-AMI trial. *EuroIntervention.* 2013;8:1134–1142.
7. Cannon CP, Gibson CM, Lambrew CT, et al. Relationship of symptom-onset-to-balloon time and door-to-balloon time with mortality in patients undergoing angioplasty for acute myocardial infarction. *JAMA.* 2000;283:2941–2947.
8. Puymirat E, Simon T, Steg PG, et al. Association of changes in clinical characteristics and management with improvement in survival among patients with ST-elevation myocardial infarction. *JAMA.* 2012;308:998–1006.
9. Invasive compared with non-invasive treatment in unstable coronary-artery disease: FRISC II prospective randomised multicentre study. FRagmin and Fast Revascularisation during InStability in Coronary artery disease Investigators. *Lancet.* 1999;354(9180):708–715.
10. Brieger D, Fox KA, Fitzgerald G, et al.; Global Registry of Acute Coronary Events Investigators. Predicting freedom from clinical events in non-ST-elevation acute coronary syndromes: The Global Registry of Acute Coronary Events. *Heart.* 2009;95:888–894.
11. Armstrong PW, Fu Y, Chang WC, et al. Acute coronary syndromes in the GUSTO-IIb trial: Prognostic insights and impact of recurrent ischemia. The GUSTO-IIb Investigators. *Circulation.* 1998;98:1860–1868.
12. Montalescot G, Dallongeville J, Van Belle E, et al. STEMI and NSTEMI: Are they so different? 1 year outcomes in acute myocardial infarction as defined by the ESC/ACC definition (the OPERA registry). *Eur Heart J.* 2007;28:1409–1417.
13. Puymirat E, Taldir G, Aissaoui N, et al. Use of invasive strategy in non-ST-segment elevation myocardial infarction is a major

determinant of improved long-term survival: FAST-MI (French Registry of Acute Coronary Syndrome). *JACC Cardiovasc Interv.* 2012;5:893–902.

14. Stone GW, Witzenbichler B, Guagliumi G, et al. Heparin plus a glycoprotein IIb/IIIa inhibitor versus bivalirudin monotherapy and paclitaxel-eluting stents versus bare-metal stents in acute myocardial infarction (HORIZONS-AMI): Final 3-year results from a multicentre, randomised controlled trials. *Lancet.* 2011;377:2193–2204.
15. Allen LA, O'Donnell CJ, Camargo CA, Jr., Giugliano RP, Lloyd-Jones DM. Comparison of long-term mortality across the spectrum of acute coronary syndromes. *Am Heart J.* 2006;151:1065–1071.
16. Hirsch A, Verouden NJ, Koch KT, et al. Comparison of long-term mortality after percutaneous coronary intervention in patients treated for acute ST-elevation myocardial infarction versus those with unstable and stable angina pectoris. *Am J Cardiol.* 2009;104:333–337.
17. Narins CR, Zareba W, Moss AJ, et al. Relationship between intermittent claudication, inflammation, thrombosis, and recurrent cardiac events among survivors of myocardial infarction. *Arch Intern Med.* 2004;164:440–446.
18. Shlipak MG, Heidenreich PA, Noguchi H, Chertow GM, Browner WS, McClellan MB. Association of renal insufficiency with treatment and outcomes after myocardial infarction in elderly patients. *Ann Intern Med.* 2002;137:555–562.
19. Anavekar NS, McMurray JJ, Velazquez EJ, et al. Relation between renal dysfunction and cardiovascular outcomes after myocardial infarction. *N Engl J Med.* 2004;351:1285–1295.
20. Pizzetti F, Turazza FM, Franzosi MG, et al. Incidence and prognostic significance of atrial fibrillation in acute myocardial infarction: The GISSI-3 data. *Heart.* 2001;86:527–532.
21. Jabre P, Jouven X, Adnet F, et al. Atrial fibrillation and death after myocardial infarction: A community study. *Circulation.* 2011;123:2094–2100.
22. Correale E, Maggioni AP, Romano S, et al. Comparison of frequency, diagnostic and prognostic significance of pericardial involvement in acute myocardial infarction treated with and without thrombolytics. Gruppo Italiano per lo Studio della Sopravvivenza nell'Infarto Miocardico (GISSI). *Am J Cardiol.* 1993;71:1377–1381.
23. Wall TC, Califf RM, Harrelson-Woodlief L, et al. Usefulness of a pericardial friction rub after thrombolytic therapy during acute myocardial infarction in predicting amount of myocardial damage. The TAMI Study Group. *Am J Cardiol.* 1990;66:1418–1421.
24. Tofler GH, Muller JE, Stone PH, et al. Pericarditis in acute myocardial infarction: Characterization and clinical significance. *Am Heart J.* 1989;117:86–92.

25. Imazio M, Negro A, Belli R, et al. Frequency and prognostic significance of pericarditis following acute myocardial infarction treated by primary percutaneous coronary intervention. *Am J Cardiol.* 2009;103:1525–1529.
26. Sugiura T, Iwasaka T, Takayama Y, et al. Factors associated with pericardial effusion in acute Q wave myocardial infarction. *Circulation.* 1990;81:477–481.
27. Figueras J, Barrabés JA, Serra V, et al. Hospital outcome of moderate to severe pericardial effusion complicating ST-elevation acute myocardial infarction. *Circulation.* 2010;122:1902–1909.
28. Patel MR, Meine TJ, Lindblad L, et al. Cardiac tamponade in the fibrinolytic era: Analysis of >100,000 patients with ST-segment elevation myocardial infarction. *Am Heart J.* 2006;151:316–322.
29. Fejka M, Dixon SR, Safian RD, et al. Diagnosis, management, and clinical outcome of cardiac tamponade complicating percutaneous coronary intervention. *Am J Cardiol.* 2002;90:1183–1186.
30. von Sohsten R, Kopistansky C, Cohen M, Kussmaul WG 3rd. Cardiac tamponade in the "new device" era: Evaluation of 6999 consecutive percutaneous coronary interventions. *Am Heart J.* 2000;140:279–283.
31. Dressler W. A post-myocardial infarction syndrome; preliminary report of a complication resembling idiopathic, recurrent, benign pericarditis. *J Am Med Assoc.* 1956;160:1379–1383.
32. Shahar A, Hod H, Barabash GM, Kaplinsky E, Motro M. Disappearance of a syndrome: Dressler's syndrome in the era of thrombolysis. *Cardiology.* 1994;85:255–258.
33. Khan AH. The postcardiac injury syndromes. *Clin Cardiol.* 1992;15:67–72.
34. Pohjola-Sintonen S, Muller JE, Stone PH, et al. Ventricular septal and free wall rupture complicating acute myocardial infarction: Experience in the Multicenter Investigation of Limitation of Infarct Size. *Am Heart J.* 1989;117:809–818.
35. Figueras J, Alcalde O, Barrabés JA, et al. Changes in hospital mortality rates in 425 patients with acute ST-elevation myocardial infarction and cardiac rupture over a 30-year period. *Circulation.* 2008;118:2783–2789.
36. Nakatsuchi Y, Minamino T, Fujii K, Negoro S. Clinicopathological characterization of cardiac free wall rupture in patients with acute myocardial infarction: Difference between early and late phase rupture. *Int J Cardiol.* 1994;47(Suppl 1):S33–S38.
37. Birnbaum Y, Fishbein MC, Blanche C, Siegel RJ. Ventricular septal rupture after acute myocardial infarction. *N Engl J Med.* 2002;347:1426–1432.
38. Crenshaw BS, Granger CB, Birnbaum Y, et al. Risk factors, angiographic patterns, and outcomes in patients with ventricular septal

defect complicating acute myocardial infarction. GUSTO-I (Global Utilization of Streptokinase and TPA for Occluded Coronary Arteries) Trial Investigators. *Circulation*. 2000;101:27- 32.

39. Radford MJ, Johnson RA, Daggett WM, Jr., et al. Ventricular septal rupture: A review of clinical and physiologic features and an analysis of survival. *Circulation*. 1981;64:545–553.

40. Skehan JD, Carey C, Norrell MS, de Belder M, Balcon R, Mills PG. Patterns of coronary artery disease in post-infarction ventricular septal rupture. *Br Heart J*. 1989;62:268–272.

41. Hayashi T, Hirano Y, Takai H, et al. Usefulness of ST-segment elevation in the inferior leads in predicting ventricular septal rupture in patients with anterior wall acute myocardial infarction. *Am J Cardiol*. 2005;96:1037–1041.

42. Picard MH, Davidoff R, Sleeper LA, et al. Echocardiographic predictors of survival and response to early revascularization in cardiogenic shock. SHOCK Trial. SHould we emergently revascularize Occluded Coronaries for cardiogenic shocK. *Circulation*. 2003;107:279–284.

43. Trichon BH, Glower DD, Shaw LK, et al. Survival after coronary revascularization, with and without mitral valve surgery, in patients with ischemic mitral regurgitation. *Circulation*. 2003;108(Suppl 1):II.103–II.110.

44. Nishimura RA, Schaff HV, Shub C, Gersh BJ, Edwards WD, Tajik AJ. Papillary muscle rupture complicating acute myocardial infarction: Analysis of 17 patients. *Am J Cardiol*. 1983;51:373–377.

45. James TN. Anatomy of the coronary arteries in health and disease. *Circulation*. 1965;32:1020–1033.

CHAPTER 4

The Role of EMS in the Triage of the ACS Patient

Jason Jones, MD, Staccie A. Allen, MSN, ARNP, EMT-P, CFRN, Christine Van Dillen, MD, Joel Rowe, MD, and Brandon Allen, MD

INTRODUCTION

For decades, "time is muscle" has been the mantra in ST elevation myocardial infarction (STEMI) evaluation and management to signify that patient benefits are exponentially increased the earlier that reperfusion therapy is initiated. Accordingly, decreasing door-to-balloon times have become a national benchmark. Every 30-minute delay has been shown to be associated with a 7.5% increase in relative risk of 1-year mortality, and overall mortality is increased by 6 patients per 1000 for every 15-minute delay past 90 minutes.[1,2]

Of course, ischemia and infarction do not begin when the patient arrives at the hospital. Emergency medical services (EMSs) help expedite care and shift the focus from *door-to-balloon* time to *symptom-to-balloon* time. Studies demonstrate that when EMS is involved in cardiac care, patients have decreased times to medical therapy and reperfusion, and decreased mortality from STEMI.[3,4,5] Furthermore, the goal of door-to-balloon time of less than 90 minutes may be achieved in as many as 86% of cases with EMS, versus 58% overall.[6,7]

Paramedics and other prehospital providers are now entrusted with a broad scope of responsibilities for the early

Acute Coronary Syndrome: Urgent and Follow-up Care © 2017
Joseph S. Alpert, Lynne T. Braun, Barbara J. Fletcher, Gerald Fletcher, Editors-in-Chief, Cardiotext Publishing, ISBN: 978-1-935395-94-2

diagnosis, treatment, and transport of patients with acute coronary syndrome (ACS). The American Heart Association (AHA) recommends that EMS personnel should be accountable for obtaining a prehospital ECG, making the diagnosis, activating the system, and deciding whether to transport the patient to a percutaneous coronary intervention (PCI) capable or non-PCI capable hospital.[8] Studies reflect that paramedics who are trained in ECG interpretation have success rates in the diagnosis of STEMI that mirror those of emergency department (ED) physicians and cardiologists.[9,10] As further justification, "Key Element #1" for hospitals seeking accreditation as Chest Pain Centers through the Society of Chest Pain Centers is ED integration with EMS.[11]

BACKGROUND

EMSs are as varied as the communities and topographies they serve. Responding agencies may range from all-volunteer units and basic first responders (including police) to critical care paramedics and flight teams capable of managing advanced interventions up to and including mechanical ventilation, vasopressors, drug infusions, broad-spectrum antibiotics, fibrinolytics, and intra-aortic balloon pumps. The federal government has created a standardized curriculum for four levels of EMS provider—first responder, emergency medical technician (EMT)-basic, EMT-intermediate, and EMT-paramedic—but there is considerable variation in the responsibilities that individual communities delegate to of each of these levels to address their local needs.[12] In general, an EMT-basic can provide first aid and perform CPR, administer an automatic external defibrillator (AED), and provide oxygen. An EMT-intermediate or paramedic can perform advanced life support, as well as advanced procedures including endotracheal intubation, ECG interpretation, and administration of medications. EMS systems are largely regulated at a state and local level, in coordination with a physician serving as medical director for each agency.

COMMUNITY OUTREACH AND PREPAREDNESS

Treatment of ACS occurs long before a patient dials 911. EMS is a public service profession, and through its unique link between patients and hospitals, it is able to provide valuable public education and outreach within the community. Common strategies include providing CPR training, raising awareness of cardiac ischemic symptoms, and stressing the importance of activating EMS. Particular attention is paid to the signs of angina, including less commonly known symptoms such as nausea, diaphoresis, dizziness, and syncope, which may occur more often in the elderly, women, and diabetics. These efforts have great potential for community benefit, as studies demonstrate that public use of EMS for chest pain ranges from only 10% to 60%, including only half of all STEMI patients.[12,13,14]

Previous EMS outreach strategies have included health fairs, workshops, news releases and print advertisements, public service announcements, and informational displays. In one well-publicized example, an intensive month-long community education effort by EMS in Wabasha County, Minnesota, resulted in a significant increase in EMS and ED usage for patients with acute chest pain.[15] A 2010 prospective randomized trial evaluated the effect of prehospital teaching on patients with recent hospital admissions. Teaching topics included recognition of ACS symptoms, activation of EMS, and the selection of a surrogate to hold the patient accountable. Among those who subsequently had chest pain requiring hospital evaluation, the intervention group had an average time from onset of symptoms to ED evaluation of 1.7 hours, versus 7.1 hours for the cohort who did not receive education.[16]

While hospitals are vigilantly trying to decrease door-to-balloon times by minutes, focusing on the education of our communities may have much more significant benefits.

DISPATCH

Dispatch services may range from a single telephone operator using flip-cards to a comprehensive telecommunications suite with sophisticated computer-aided dispatch (CAD) programs integrated with the entire healthcare system.[17] In general, emergency medical dispatchers are professionals who receive extensive training on the evidence-based protocols that help them determine a caller's level of acuity. A majority of EMS systems use a "multitiered response" to dispatch more than one type of resource to time-sensitive calls. The dispatch center serves as the first tier by answering calls and activating resources, a rapid response team (which may not be an ambulance) represents the second tier, and a transport ambulance represents the third tier. Priority symptoms such as chest pain and respiratory distress often warrant a dispatcher to request a "dual-hot" response. The resources utilized for a "dual-hot" activation usually include two units with lights-and-sirens traveling urgently, with at least one unit capable of providing advanced life support. Increasingly, emergency medical dispatchers are also trained to instruct callers to self-administer aspirin and to perform CPR if indicated.[18] A 2001 study by Rea et al. showed that dispatcher-instructed CPR is successful and increases survival rates in cardiac arrest.[19]

ON-SCENE CARE

When a paramedic arrives at the scene of an emergency call, he or she will perform a primary survey to evaluate the patient's airway, breathing, and circulation and measure vital signs. At that time, he or she will perform a focused history and physical examination. From the information obtained, the paramedic's duties are two-fold. He or she must determine the most life-threatening conditions that may be present, and must select the medical protocol that best reflects the patient's presentation. Paramedics are well trained in these tasks, and the national EMT-paramedic core curriculum includes considerable teaching on cardiac anatomy and pathophysiology, typical and atypical symptoms of angina, ECG interpretation, and appropriate treatment in emergent cardiac care.[12]

For patients with presentations suspicious for ACS, performing a 12-lead ECG within 5 minutes of patient contact becomes the priority, and further history and physical exam may be abbreviated or deferred. Several studies have demonstrated that paramedics with ECG training have success rates in detecting STEMI that mirror those of emergency physicians and cardiologists, with specificity ranging from 91% to 100%.[12] If an STEMI is present, the paramedic's priority is then to notify the receiving hospital immediately to activate the cardiac catheterization laboratory. If STEMI is not detected but high concern for ACS is present, the paramedic may perform a right-sided ECG to evaluate for a posterior MI.[18]

EMS systems vary in who is responsible for STEMI recognition and cardiac catheterization lab activation. Many systems rely on paramedic interpretation alone for STEMI alert activation, while others rely on computer-assisted interpretation, interpretation by an ED physician or cardiologist after digital transmission, or a combination of these methods. Nevertheless, AHA guidelines recommend paramedic responsibility, stating "EMS personnel should be accountable for obtaining a prehospital ECG, making the diagnosis, activating the system, and deciding whether to transport the patient to a PCI-capable or non-PCI capable hospital."[8]

One issue complicating paramedic ECG interpretation is the presence of so-called mimics of STEMI, including pericarditis and left bundle branch block (LBBB). Medical directors and hospital representatives must determine whether these false positives are acceptable. Medical directors may also consider whether providing specialized training to paramedics (such as the Sgarbossa criteria for LBBB) is feasible. Nevertheless, EMS performance of a 12-lead ECG remains a class I AHA recommendation.[8] Prehospital ECGs often detect ischemic changes that may resolve prior to hospital arrival or evolve into appreciable ischemia or infarction. One study determined increased sensitivity for an acute cardiac event by comparing prehospital and hospital-based ECGs.[20]

Once an ECG has been performed and interpreted, EMS culture has shifted to a "scoop and run" strategy for patients with symptoms consistent with ACS. A profound emphasis has been placed on minimizing time on scene, responding "hot" with lights and sirens if the system permits, and performing further interventions *en route* rather than at the scene. These interventions typically follow AHA guidelines and include establishing intravenous access and administering nonenteric aspirin, oxygen (if oxygen saturation is ≤ 94%), nitroglycerin (if an inferior or posterior infarct is not evident), morphine for pain refractory to nitroglycerin, and crystalloid fluids (for posterior or inferior infarcts).[18] The patient is typically kept on a cardiac monitor and evaluated for dynamic changes on telemetry or changes in vital signs. Some advanced rescue units may also administer heparin, clopidogrel (Plavix), and/or glycoprotein IIB/IIIA antagonists.[21]

Fibrinolytic medications remain an area of controversy in the prehospital setting. AHA guidelines recommend administering fibrinolytics within 30 minutes of patient contact if the time from first medical contact to PCI will exceed 120 minutes.[18] Fibrinolytic therapy for STEMI in the prehospital setting was introduced in Jerusalem, Israel, in 1985 and has been employed to varying degrees since that time.[21] Existing evidence demonstrates a survival benefit for prehospital rather than hospital administration of fibrinolytics in STEMI, with one study demonstrating a 15% relative risk reduction in early mortality.[22] This may be a critical consideration for EMS agencies with long transport times, as 1 patient in 5 lives more than 1 hour away from a PCI-capable center.[23] The AHA recommends that agencies administering pre-hospital fibrinolytics have "protocols using fibrinolytic checklists, 12-lead ECG acquisition and interpretation, experience in advanced life support, communication with the receiving institution, a medical director with training and experience in STEMI management, and continuous quality improvement."[18]

THE EMS-HOSPITAL INTERFACE

The rescue unit's ultimate destination is the hospital best able to care for the patient, and it is the paramedic's role to provide an accurate report to the ED staff of his or her assessment and care. Once these two elements of prehospital care are achieved, care of the patient is transferred to the hospital team, and the rescue unit notifies dispatch that it is available for further emergency calls. In an ideal STEMI scenario, the cardiac catheterization laboratory is already prepared for the patient, and the ED and cardiology teams are present for the patient's arrival. However, EMS agencies, EMS medical directors, and hospital officials have several important decisions that determine the flow of a patient's arrival.

EMS medical directors typically create a destination protocol for ACS and STEMI patients, according to AHA guidelines, so that EMS providers deliver patients to the most appropriate facility. A major consideration is whether rescue units should bypass hospitals without PCI capability to take patients to those with PCI capability. One study demonstrated that even among patients who lived closer to a non-PCI-capable hospital, three-fourths would experience a less-than-30-minute delay if routed to a PCI-capable hospital.[23] Another major decision is whether the rescue unit should deliver the STEMI patient to the ED or directly to the cardiac catheterization lab. This decreases door-to-balloon times, but may place unstable patients or those with other life-threatening conditions in the catheterization lab rather than an ED resuscitation room. Lastly, EMS agencies and hospitals must determine who is able to activate the cardiac catheterization laboratory. Options include automated activation by EMS, activation by the ED team upon patient arrival, and/or activation only by a cardiologist. These system-based decisions can greatly impact the flow of a patient's care, and without interdisciplinary communication have the potential to result in increased morbidity and mortality.

REFERENCES

1. De Luca G, Suryapranata H, Ottervanger JP, Antman EM. Time delay to treatment and mortality in primary angioplasty for acute myocardial infarction: Every minute of delay counts. *Circulation.* 2004;109(10):1223–1225.
2. McNamara RL, Wang Y, Herrin J, et al. Effect of door-to-balloon time on mortality in patients with ST-segment elevation myocardial infarction. *J Amer Coll Cardio.* 2006;47(11):2180–2186.
3. Hutchings CB, Mann NC, Daya M, et al. Patients with chest pain calling 9-1-1 or self-transporting to reach definitive care: Which mode is quicker? *Am Heart J.* 2004;147(1):35–41.
4. van't Hof AW, Rasoul S, van de Wetering H, et al. Feasibility and benefit of prehospital diagnosis, triage, and therapy by paramedics only in patients who are candidates for primary angioplasty for acute myocardial infarction. *Am Heart J.* 2006;151(6):1255.
5. Patel M, Dunford JV, Aguilar S, et al. Pre-hospital electrocardiography by emergency medical personnel: Effects on scene and transport times for chest pain and ST-segment elevation myocardial infarction patients. *J Am Coll Cardio.* 2012;60(9):806–811.
6. Rokos IC, French WJ, Koenig WJ, et al. Integration of pre-hospital electrocardiograms and ST-elevation myocardial infarction receiving center (SRC) networks: Impact on door-to-balloon times across 10 independent regions. *JACC Cardiovasc Interv.* 2009;2(4):339–346.
7. Daudelin DH, Sayah AJ, Kwong M, et al. Improving use of prehospital 12-lead ECG for early identification and treatment of acute coronary syndrome and ST-elevation myocardial infarction. *Circ Cardiovasc Qual Outcomes.* 2010;3(3):316–323.
8. O'Gara P, Kushner F, Ascheim D, et al. 2013 ACCF/AHA guideline for the management of ST-elevation myocardial infarction:

A report of the American College of Cardiology Foundation/ American Heart Association Task Force on Practice Guidelines. *Circulation*. 2012;127(4):e362–e425.

9. Ferguson JD, Brady WJ, Perron AD, et al. The prehospital 12-lead electrocardiogram: Impact on management of the out-of-hospital acute coronary syndrome patient. *Am J Emerg Med*. 2003;21(2): 136–142.
10. Foster DB, Dufendach JH, Barkdoll CM, Mitchell BK. Prehospital recognition of AMI using independent nurse/paramedic 12-lead ECG evaluation: Impact on in-hospital times to thrombolysis in a rural community hospital. *Am J Emerg Med*. 1994;12(1): 25–31.
11. Miracle K. The role and involvement of EMS: Strategies for streamlined STEMI & stroke care. *Cath Lab Digest*. 2011;19(7):38–40.
12. Ting HH, Krumholz HM, Bradley EH, et al. Implementation and integration of prehospital ECGs into systems of care for acute coronary syndrome: A scientific statement from the American Heart Association Interdisciplinary Council on Quality of Care and Outcomes Research, Emergency Cardiovascular Care Committee, Council on Cardiovascular Nursing, and Council on Clinical Cardiology. *Circulation*. 2008;118(10):1066–1079.
13. Garvey JL, MacLeod BA, Sopko G, et al. Pre-hospital 12-lead electrocardiography programs—A call for implementation by emergency medical services systems providing advanced life support—National Heart Attack Alert Program (NHAAP) Coordinating Committee; National Heart, Lung, and Blood Institute (NHLBI); National Institutes of Health. *J Am Coll Cardiol*. 2006;47(3):485–491.
14. Matthews R, Peterson ED, Li S, et al. Use of emergency medical service transport among patients with ST-segment-elevation myocardial infarction: Findings from the National Cardiovascular Data Registry Acute Coronary Treatment Intervention Outcomes Network Registry-Get With The Guidelines. *Circulation*. 2011;124(2):154–163.
15. Wright RS, Kopecky SL, Timm M, et al. Impact of community-based education on health care evaluation in patients with acute chest pain syndromes: The Wabasha Heart Attack Team (WHAT) project. *Fam Pract*. 2001;18(5):537–539.
16. Mooney M, McKee G, Fealy G, et al. A randomized controlled trial to reduce prehospital delay time in patients with acute coronary syndrome (ACS). *J Emerg Med*. 2014;46(4):495–506.
17. Overton J. Saving lives begins here. JEMS supplemental (Data Drives Care). 2014;6–9.
18. O'Connor RE, Brady W, Brooks SC, et al. Part 10: Acute coronary syndromes: 2010 American Heart Association Guidelines for Cardiopulmonary Resuscitation and Emergency Cardiovascular Care. *Circulation*. 2010;122(18 Suppl 3):S787–817.

19. Rea T, Eisenberg M, Culley L, Becker L. Dispatcher-assisted cardiopulmonary resuscitation and survival in cardiac arrest. *Circulation.* 2001;104:2513–2516.
20. Kudenchuk PJ, Maynard C, Cobb LA, et al. Utility of the prehospital electrocardiogram in diagnosing acute coronary syndromes: The myocardial infarction triage and intervention (MITI) project. *J Am Coll Cardio.* 1998;32(1):17–27.
21. Verheugt F. Reperfusion therapy starts in the ambulance. *Circulation.* 2006;113(20):2377–2379.
22. Morrison LJ, Verbeek PR, McDonald AC, Sawadsky BV, Cook DJ. Mortality and prehospital thrombolysis for acute myocardial infarction. *JAMA.* 2000;283(20):2686–2692.
23. Nallamothu B, Bates E, Wang Y, Bradley E, Krumholz H. Driving times and distances to hospitals with percutaneous coronary intervention in the United States. *Circulation.* 2006;113(9):1189–1195.

CHAPTER 5

Evaluation and Treatment of the Acute Coronary Syndrome Patient in the Emergency Department

Preeti Jois, MD, Samantha Noah, RN, and Robert S. Svingos, PharmD

BACKGROUND

In the most recent publication by the National Hospital Ambulatory Medical Care Survey, "chest pain" received credit as the second-most common reason for a visit to the emergency department (ED). Even more remarkable is the finding that nonischemic heart disease, chest pain, and ischemic heart disease were the top three leading principal hospital discharge diagnoses for the same ED visits survey.[1] Overall, from 1999 to 2008, the percentage of ED visits for which chest pain was the primary complaint decreased by 10% and the percentage of ED visits for chest pain resulting in a diagnosis of acute coronary syndrome (ACS) decreased by 44.9%. In the period from 1999 to 2008, the percentage of chest pain visits triaged as "immediate" or "emergent" (defined as *should be seen within 14 minutes*) decreased by 12.4%. Nonetheless, in this same time period, it was noted that patients with chest pain were more likely to die,

Acute Coronary Syndrome: Urgent and Follow-up Care © 2017
Joseph S. Alpert, Lynne T. Braun, Barbara J. Fletcher, Gerald Fletcher, Editors-in-Chief,
Cardiotext Publishing, ISBN: 978-1-935395-94-2

be admitted to the hospital, or be transferred to another facility compared to visits for abdominal pain or other symptoms.[2]

Patients presenting to the ED for evaluation of "chest pain" pose a complex and challenging problem for the ED physician. They account for approximately 6% to 8% of all ED visits nationally, or approximately 6–8 million patients. The sheer volume of patients creates a burden on ED providers and the acute healthcare system. The inappropriate or inadvertent discharge of the ACS patient is a constant worry for the ED physician/healthcare provider (HCP). Although current American College of Emergency Physician (ACEP) guidelines exist to assist with the appropriate and timely triage and evaluation of these patients, historically up to 8% of patients with acute myocardial infarction (AMI) or ACS have been discharged home.[3] Recent data suggest that close to 2.1% of patients with AMI receive the wrong diagnosis and are discharged home, leading to a 30-day mortality rate of 9.1%.[4] In the clinical setting, this has had the unfortunate effect of putting large numbers of otherwise low-risk chest pain patients through formal diagnostic testing for ACS. In this particular population of patients, prolonged evaluations have led to false-positive findings, unnecessary downstream procedures, and rising healthcare costs.[5] Current efforts to improve upon this finding include 1) focus on risk stratification of patients presenting with chest pains—evaluating the likelihood that the current presentation is due to acute MI and 2) rapid assessment for a major adverse cardiac events (MACEs)—evaluating underlying risk for non-ST elevation myocardial infarction (NSTEMI) and unstable angina.[6]

APPROACH TO THE ED PATIENT WITH CHEST PAIN

The initial evaluation of the patient presenting to the ED with a complaint of chest pain includes a thorough patient history, physical exam, and an ECG.

Electrocardiogram

Guidelines established in 2000 and reinforced in current documents recommend that an ECG be obtained within 10 minutes of a patient presenting with a complaint of chest pain.[7] Diercks et al. showed a worsened outcome with delays greater than 10 minutes to an initial ECG, especially in patients presenting with STEMI.[8] ED physicians, advanced registered nurse practitioners, and physician assistants are closely scrutinized by another tracked metric, ECG-to-doctor time.

The ECG provides a sound objective risk stratification tool to rapidly ascertain the presence of STEMI or other findings consistent with an ACS. The presence of ischemic changes identifies a patient at high-risk of ACS. Unfortunately, a seemingly normal ECG, or one without obvious markers of a possible ACS, may miss the patient with underlying unstable angina, especially if the ECG is obtained when the patient is pain-free. While the ECG may help rapidly identify the patient with ACS, it may overlook the patient with yet undiagnosed coronary artery disease (CAD). In the ED setting, it is important to make this distinction, especially given the large number of patients who present for chest pain evaluation. The explicit goal of chest pain evaluation in the ED is to rapidly recognize and treat the patient with current ACS, not to necessarily identify all potential patients with underlying CAD not presently manifesting as ACS.

Key Nursing Intervention

ECG

Although physicians are responsible for prescribing and directing care for patients who present to the ED with ACS, nurses play an extremely important role in making sure that practice guidelines are met. Perhaps the most important aspect of triaging any patient presenting to the ED with possible ACS is obtaining a 12-lead ECG. The ECG is the cornerstone tool used to assess chest pain patients in the ED. Triage nurses have three basic responsibilities when it comes to obtaining an ECG. First, the ECG must be completed in less than 10 minutes of arrival time. Second, ECG electrodes must be placed accurately and consistently. Third, prior ECGs for comparison should be obtained if possible.[9] Achievement of these goals will likely require having a staff member in triage whose sole responsibility is to obtain an ECG on all patients who present with a chief complaint above the belt line. There is no need to wait for registration or triage to obtain an ECG. Studies have shown that waiting for triage or registration increases door-to-ECG time, which ultimately increases door-to-balloon (D2B) time.[10] Proper lead placement is essential for obtaining an accurate ECG. Placing all ten electrodes in their predetermined location is not time-consuming if you are familiar with the landmarks for lead placement. There are six precordial leads (V_1–V_6) and four limb leads (LA, RA, LL, RL). For placement of the precordial chest leads, it is best to start with V_1, which is placed at the fourth intercostal space (ICS) on the right sternal border. It is possible to palpate the ICSs on most patients, even those who are obese. On the rare occasion that the ICS cannot be palpated, the location of V_1 can be estimated based on the location of the clavicle. Appropriate placement of V_1 is essential because placement of the rest of your precordial leads will be based on this. Finding the fourth ICS is done by first palpating the suprasternal notch, or jugular notch. The suprasternal notch is found at the top of the sternum, between the two clavicular notches. Now move your finger down to find the sternal angle, or the angle of Louis, which feels like a bony horizontal ridge. Once you have located the sternal angle, move your fingers to the patient's right, and you will be at the second ICS. Now palpate downward two more spaces and place V_1 in its proper location.

V_2 is placed at the fourth ICS on the left sternal border. You will skip V_3 placement for now. Place V_4 at the fifth ICS at the left midclavicular line. For many male and nonobese patients, this is in line with the nipple. Now place V_3 directly between V_2 and V_4. V_5 is also at the fifth ICS, level with V_4, at the left anterior axillary line. V_6, again, is placed at the fifth ICS, this time at the left mid axillary line.[11] Placement of V_6 will require asking the patient to move his or her arm out of the way. Proper lead placement on female patients can be challenging due to breast tissue. Explain what you are doing to the patient. At that point, you can ask the patient to lift her breast, or use the back of your left hand to move the breast tissue out of the way. Movement of excess soft tissue must be done in order to obtain an accurate ECG.

The four remaining limb leads can be attached anywhere on the arms or legs, as long as they are not touching the thorax. Remember to avoid placing any lead over a bony prominence because this may cause unnecessary artifact.[12] Whenever possible, bring the patient's most recent prior ECG with you, along with the current ECG, to the physician or HCP who will be evaluating them. This allows for an appropriate comparison.

Triage

While the ECG is an essential tool in the initial triage of chest pain patients in the ED, it should not be viewed in isolation from the patient's history and current clinical state. Obtaining an accurate patient history in triage will augment the accuracy of the physician's diagnosis. The medical history obtained in triage should focus on accurate pain assessment. When seconds count during triage, the PQRST mnemonic for pain assessment[13] offers a simple, reliable, and consistent approach to the best documentation of what the patient is experiencing.

1) P—provoking and palliating factors. What brings the pain on? What makes the pain worse? What can you

do to alleviate the pain? Does the pain get worse with activity, movement, or deep inspiration? Does it get better with rest?

2) Q—quality of the pain. Ask the patient to use descriptive words to tell you about the pain. Examples include stabbing, crushing, burning, and nagging.
3) R—region/radiation/reproducibility. Describe the region, or location, of the pain. Ask the patient to point to the location where the pain is at its worst. Does the pain radiate anywhere? Can I reproduce the pain by pressing or palpating here?
4) S—severity and associated symptoms. Pain severity is subjective, but the most accurate way to assess it is to use a 0–10 pain scale. Ask the patient to rate the pain they are currently experiencing on a scale from 0 to 10. Are you experiencing any other symptoms with the pain? Nausea or vomiting? Fever or chills? Shortness of breath? Sweating? Cough? Palpitations?
5) T—timing. When did the pain start? How long did it last? Are you still experiencing the pain? What were you doing when the pain started? Is the pain constant, or does it come and go? Did the pain start suddenly, or did it develop over a period of time?

In addition to a thorough pain assessment in triage, it is imperative to obtain a complete set of vital signs. A team approach will improve overall timing. For example, while a nurse is obtaining a pain assessment and patient history, a second staff member is having a physician review the ECGs and is getting a complete set of vital signs. Other patient history information that is important to document in the triage note includes current medications, allergies, known risk factors for CAD such as diabetes and smoking history, history of previous admissions for chest pain or ACS, past history of intervention for CAD/ACS, including percutaneous coronary intervention (PCI) or coronary artery bypass graft surgery (CABG), and known cerebral vascular or peripheral vascular disease.[9]

All possible ACS patients should be brought to a monitored treatment room immediately upon completion of triage. While the physician is examining the patient and taking a more detailed medical history, the nurse facilitates diagnosis by establishing at least one large bore (18 g or larger if possible) IV and taking blood samples for serum biomarkers and other labs. Draw labs according to your particular institution's protocol. Some hospitals may require the blood to be transported to the laboratory, while others perform blood tests at the bedside by a qualified nurse.[9] Again, a team approach is key. While the nurse establishes IV access and drawing blood, second and third staff members undress the patient, attach the leads from the bedside monitor, and initiate supplemental oxygen as directed by the physician.

Patient History

The patient history is one of the most crucial pieces of the approach to the ED patient with chest pain. Characteristics of the pain—onset, associated symptoms, alleviating and aggravating factors, and caliber/quality of pain—are each important clues. Some patients may not actually have "pain" in the traditional sense, instead classifying symptoms as a pressure, tightness, or discomfort. Searching for underlying risk factors such as diabetes, hypertension, family history, and personal history of prior MI or stroke will allow more optimal quantification and risk stratification for immediate acute events. In the ED patient, the three most important risk factors predictive of an ACS event are 1) personal history of CAD, 2) advanced age, and 3) gender.[14,15]

Physical Exam

Vital signs provide important clues as to the etiology of the patient's chest pain. Fever and tachycardia will often lead the practitioner down one differential diagnosis pathway, whereas the presence of hypotension and bradycardia may signal the presence of cardiovascular deterioration due to ischemia, infarction, or pump failure. The patient's general appearance will add further details to possible underlying etiologies—for example, pallor, somonolence, and diaphoresis will convey information to support presenting vital signs.

When the situation allows, it is important to perform a focused, detailed physical exam. In the case of a patient in extremis, the priorities will be focused on management of airway, breathing, and circulation (ABC). However, once ABCs have been established and stabilized, the practitioner should spend time at the bedside gathering useful information from the physical exam. Distended neck veins and muffled heart tones will suggest pericardial fluid collection causing chest pain, whereas the presence of a new murmur may suggest faulty valvular mechanism, a ruptured papillary muscle, or other potential mechanical complication of an acute ischemic event. The auscultation of pulmonary rales and the presence of bilateral lower extremity edema will disclose information about the patient's overall volume and cardiac function status. The finding of an acute herpetic zoster rash overlying the left chest wall is an example of a noncardiac reason for a patient's chest pain.

STEMI PATIENT IN THE ED

Initial Approach

As previously discussed, the most important diagnostic tool to identify a STEMI patient is the ECG. The 2013 Focused Update to the STEMI guidelines stress the importance of rapid recognition and timely reperfusion of patients with STEMI.[16] As noted within the updated guidelines, only a minority of U.S. hospitals have the capability to perform primary PCI, and any delay in time to reperfusion therapy after hospital arrival has significant implications for in-hospital mortality. The 2013 committee actually returns to the initial principal from the 2004 guideline update stating, "the appropriate and timely use of some form of reperfusion therapy is likely more important than the choice of therapy."[17]

Door-to-Device Time

In 2006, the American College of Cardiology launched the D2B initiative to improve door-to-device times in patients presenting with STEMI. In 2008, the D2B Alliance met its primary goal, showing that participating PCI-capable hospitals had achieved a D2B time on average of ≤90 minutes in at least 75% of nontransferred patients with STEMI.[18] The D2B time interval comprises three key components: 1) door-to-ECG time, 2) ECG-to-catheterization laboratory (cath lab) time, and 3) cath lab arrival-to-device time.[19] The first two components are ED specific and can have important impact on the "upstream" time required to get a patient to the cath lab.

In a different era of healthcare, the concept of an ED physician activating the cath lab/PCI team would have been nonexistent. A statement paper published in 1995 cited appropriate competencies for ECG interpretation—minimum training, education, and experiences to competently perform ECG reading were elaborated.[20] A subsequent response paper appropriately cited multiple studies showing that emergency physicians accurately interpret ECGs in the patient care interval, often without the benefit of prior ECG tracings.[21] Fortunately, years of improved collaboration between the specialties as well as improved teaching, training, and clinical practice in emergency medicine residency programs has shifted the onus of STEMI ECG recognition to the ED provider, to include emergency medical services (EMSs) teams if they are the first to obtain an ECG in the field.

Recent studies of the top-performing PCI hospitals show common driving forces which lead to improved door-to-device times and patient outcomes. The culture in these hospitals is centered on a collaborative approach, a dedicated multidisciplinary team committed to improved D2B times, innovative protocols, and data collection tools to monitor progress, identify setbacks, and create successes.[22] These centers have created key processes to replicate and standardize their evaluation and treatment of STEMI patients, often utilizing a checklist. Whether STEMI diagnosis is made by the EMS crew at the initial scene response or by the ED physician after interpreting the presenting ECG, the PCI system is activated with one central page. The entire STEMI care team is provided with timely feedback on the case, thereby allowing for detailed evaluation of the process.

Optimal ED Management

Initial ED evaluation of any acute patient is the same: airway, breathing, circulation, and disability, exposure. In the case of the STEMI patient, a full set of vital signs is obtained as the patient is undressed, placed in a gown on the gurney, and hooked up to continuous cardiac monitoring. The patient is given supplemental oxygen in the appropriately deemed fashion if needed (i.e., nasal cannula, nonrebreather, and orotracheal intubation) and intravenous (IV) fluids are started. Medications are administered in compliance with the ACCF/AHA guidelines on STEMI management.

Initial Pharmacotherapy for Suspected ACS

Initial antiplatelet therapy with aspirin should be considered in all patients presenting to the ED with suspected ACS, regardless of where on the spectrum each patient resides. Aspirin has long been a cornerstone of drug therapy in patients with ACS. Its mortality benefit has been previously published in a myriad of studies, which, for conciseness, will not be elaborated upon in this chapter. The 2013 ACC/AHA STEMI guidelines[16] recommend nonenteric coated aspirin 162–325 mg, chewed, as soon as possible unless a severe allergy is known.

Anti-anginal therapy may also be given in the form of sublingual (SL) or IV nitroglycerin if the patient is hemodynamically stable. Nitroglycerin 0.4 mg SL should be administered initially for angina symptoms. A dose may be given every 5 minutes for a maximum of three doses. For persistent angina in the setting of elevated blood pressure and/or heart failure symptoms, IV nitroglycerin (Tridil gtt) is preferred. Consider avoiding the use of nitroglycerin in patients with suspected right ventricular (RV) infarction, as these patients may deteriorate quickly after the administration of venodilating agents. The prudent practitioner should also inquire about the recent use of erectile dysfunction medications, particularly phosphodiesterase type 5 (PDE5) inhibitors. Nitrates are contraindicated in patients who have taken sildenafil or vardenafil within the previous 24 hours, or tadalafil within 48 hours.

Additional analgesia should be considered in patients with ongoing angina who fail to respond to nitrates. Morphine sulfate is the preferred analgesic in ACS, particularly if anxiety or pulmonary edema are present. The effective dose varies between patients, but typically ranges between 2 and 8 mg IV. Safe administration should occur in a step-wise fashion beginning with 2–4 mg IV initially, with at least 10 minutes between subsequent doses. This time period allows for the full analgesic effects to be realized, while also minimizing the potential for opioid-induced respiratory depression. Existing literature suggests the use of nonsteroidal anti-inflammatory drugs and cyclooxygenase II inhibitors may be associated with increased morbidity and mortality. Based on their potential for harm, these medication classes are contraindicated in patients with suspected or confirmed ACS. A complete discussion of the pharmacologic management of ACS patients is presented in Chapter 7.

Team Principles

The primary goal when administering therapy for ACS is to stop ischemia and restore flow to the myocardium. Medications will be ordered by the physician and administered by the nurse. Some institutions may require verification by a pharmacist. In this case, the pharmacist should be in the ED, preferably at the bedside. Nurses should have a clear understanding of why they are administering each medication, and how the medication may affect the patient. This information should be verbalized to the patient or family in manner that is clear and easy to understand.

All medications should be documented according to hospital protocol, being sure to adhere to the five rights. When administering nitroglycerin and morphine specifically for pain management, it is imperative that heart rate, blood pressure, and subjective pain scale be documented before and after administration of every dose.

Transferring the STEMI Patient

In-House—ED to Cath Lab

In PCI-capable facilities, a "STEMI-Activation" plan is critical in providing evidence-based care to the patient. As discussed elsewhere in this chapter, prehospital ECGs and notification to the receiving center along with activation of the cath lab team are among the important factors to shorten time to reperfusion. Rapid identification and management of the STEMI patient in the ED, along with a "one-call" notification process from the ED, will further expedite care from the department to the cath lab. Collaboration between care providers in the ED and the cath lab are also key components in the timely transfer of patient care. Quality assurance and rapid feedback programs will help ensure maintenance and improvement of programs.[22,23]

Transfer—Referring ED to Accepting Cath Lab

EDs and hospitals should have protocols in place to easily identify those patients who meet criteria that would suggest a benefit from transfer to a PCI-capable facility. The list of patients who meet this criteria can be found in the 2010 AHA guidelines for cardiopulmonary resuscitation and emergency cardiovascular care services.[24] The ACC/AHA recommends a door-to-departure time of <30 minutes.

Team-Based Approach

The physician will be responsible for contacting the cardiology or cardiac cath lab team. The nurse is responsible for communicating all necessary information to the receiving team. For patients not going directly to the cath lab, the report may be called to an intensive care unit or chest pain unit. The nurse should know and be able to immediately share information about the patient's medical history, presenting symptoms and pain assessment, vital signs, ECG assessment, medications that have been administered, and response to the medications. Calling report should in no way delay transfer to the cardiac cath lab, and may be given at the bedside if necessary. A team approach is still necessary, even though the patient may have been stabilized. While the nurse is communicating report to the receiving team, another ED staff member is packing the patient's clothes and belongings according to hospital policy, placing the patient on a portable monitor, and securing a full oxygen tank for transport. In some facilities, members of the cath lab team may be assisting with these duties.

NSTEMI AND UNSTABLE ANGINA PATIENT IN THE ED

Contrary to popular thought, the majority of patients who present to the ED with chest pain and are deemed to have

ACS and go on to have PCI in the hospital are actually either NSTEMI or unstable angina patients. NSTEMI patients tend to present with high-risk factors including female gender, history of diabetes mellitus, prior MI or PCI, prior CABG, and prior stroke. Additionally, NSTEMI patients face morbidity and mortality rates approaching their STEMI counterparts, as shown in the hospital GRACE Registry.[25]

Particularly at-risk are ACS patients who present without chest pain. Data from the National Registry of Myocardial Infarction report that nearly half of NSTEMI patients do not have chest pain when first seen.[26] In general, these patients tend to be older, more often female, and have a history of diabetes or heart failure. These patients also wait longer to present to the hospital for evaluation, on average 8 hours after their initial symptoms.[27] Compared with ACS patients who present with chest pain, ACS patients without pain are less likely to receive a diagnoses of MI at time of admission (22% pain-free ACS vs. 50% pain associated with ACS). Subsequently this population is also less likely to receive primary PCI, aspirin, beta blockers, and/or heparin. The combination of all these factors portends higher in-hospital mortality, with rates approaching 23%, compared with 9% for ACS patients with chest pain. Morbidity rates are also high in this at-risk group, with higher rates of congestive heart failure, cardiogenic shock, atrial fibrillation, ventricular fibrillation (VF)/ventricular tachycardia (VT), and acute renal failure.[28]

As we have seen previously, many hospitals have well instituted programs to provide timely care and intervention to the STEMI patient. The NSTEMI ACS patient provides an important opportunity for the use of guideline-recommended care. Every 10% increase in adherence to guideline-based therapies leads to a 10% reduction in in-hospital mortality.[29] A multidisciplinary approach clearly provides multiple benefits. This idea has become so important that the 2011 ACCF/AHA guidelines recommended quality initiative programs (ACTION-GWTG:

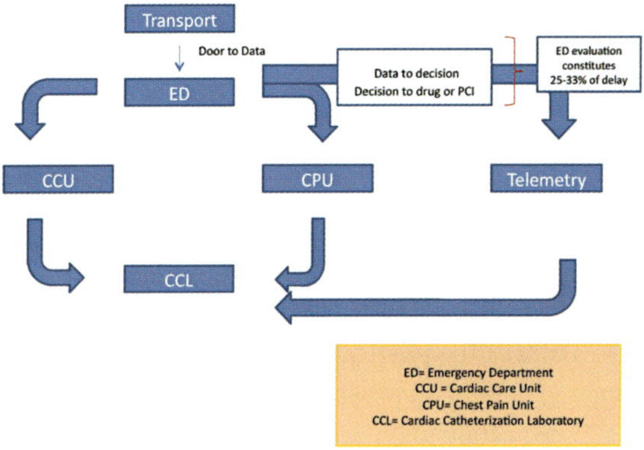

Figure 5.1

A team-based approach for patients with unstable angina/NSTEMI.

Acute Coronary Treatment and Intervention Outcomes Network—Get With the Guidelines) to improve overall patient care.[27] (See **Figure 5.1**.)

THE "LOW-TO-MODERATE RISK" CHEST PAIN PATIENT IN THE ED

Although chest pain is a frequent presenting complaint, only about 25% of all patients presenting with chest pain actually have ACS (unstable angina, NSTEMI, or STEMI).[30] The dilemma lies in the evaluation of the other 75% of those presenting with "chest pain." Studies have shown that a small percentage of these patients are at very low risk (<5%) for MACE. Barring the presence of obvious symptoms, and with a normal physical exam and an ECG without abnormalities, it is suggested that these patients could be discharged safely from the ED. Their expected outpatient 30-day MACE risk is 2.5%.[31] Interestingly, in a recent global survey of 1029 emergency physicians, there were two peaks in the distribution of "acceptable miss rate for MACE," 0.1% and 1%. This suggests that a small miss rate is acceptable to most ED physicians with the caveat that diagnostic strategies reach sensitivities of 99% or higher for AMI or chest-pain related MACE.[32]

ROLE OF THE CHEST PAIN OBSERVATION UNIT

Many EDs have the physical space and staffing required for an annexed chest pain observation unit. Chest pain units do require a dedication to implementation, staffing, and training, and these may not be ideal in every ED setting. Nonetheless, for the intermediate-risk patient presenting with chest pain, this type of unit or a process facilitating 24-hour observation admission to the hospital can be beneficial.[33] Chest pain observation protocols are designed to provide a rapid system of assessment including history and physical exam, an observation period, serial biomarkers, and serial ECGs. Several randomized trials have shown that utilization of protocol-driven chest pain units may improve accuracy in identifying patients who would benefit from hospital admission and further cardiac evaluation, by reducing overall rate of hospital admissions, healthcare costs and length of stay.[34,35]

REFERENCES

1. *National Hospital Ambulatory Medical Care Survey: 2010 Emergency Department Summary Tables.* Centers for Disease Control and Prevention, National Center for Health Statistics, Hyattsville, MD. http://www.cdc.gov/nchs/data/ahcd/nhamcs_emergency/2010_ed_web_tables.pdf. Accessed December 8, 2015.
2. Bhuiya FA, Pitts SR, McCaig LF. Emergency department visits for chest pain and abdominal pain: United States 1999-2008. *NCHS Data Brief.* 2010;43:1–8.
3. Lee TH, Rouan GW, Weisberg MC, et al. Clinical characteristics and natural history of patients with acute myocardial infarction sent home from the emergency room. *Am J Cardiol.* 1987;60:219–224.

4. Schull MJ, Vermeulen MJ, Stukel TA. The risk of missed diagnosis of acute myocardial infarction associated with emergency department volume. *Ann Emerg Med.* 2006;48:647–655.
5. Pines JM, Szyld D. Risk tolerance for the exclusion of potentially life-threatening diseases in the ED. *Am J Emerg Med.* 2007;25:540–544.
6. Amsterdam EA, Wenger NK, Brindis RG, et al. 2014 AHA/ACC guideline for the management of patients with non-ST-elevation acute coronary syndromes: A report of the American College of Cardiology/American Heart Association Task Force on Practice Guidelines. *J Am Coll Cardiol.* 2014;64(24):e139–e228.
7. Braunwald E, Antman EM, Beasley JW, et al. ACC/AHA guidelines for the management of patients with unstable angina and non-ST-segment elevation myocardial infarction. A report of the American College of Cardiology/American Heart Association Task Force on Practice Guidelines (Committee on the Management of Patients with Unstable Angina). *J Am Coll Cardiol.* 2000;36(3):970–1062.
8. Diercks DB, Kirk JD, Lindsell CJ, et al. Door-to-ECG time in patients with chest pain presenting to the ED. *Am J Emerg Med.* 2006;24:1–7.
9. Siebens K, Moons P, DeGeest S, et al. The role of nurses in a chest pain unit. *Eur J Cardiovasc Nurs.* 2007;6:265–272.
10. Phelan MP, Glauser J, Smith E, et al. Improving emergency department door-to-electrocardiogram time in ST segment elevation myocardial infarction. *Crit Pathw Cardiol.* 2009;8(3):119–121.
11. Srivastava S, Ball L, Smith R. ECG recording in obese patients. [Letter.] *BMJ.* 2006;333:1060. doi: http://dx.doi.org/10.1136/bmj.333.7577.1060
12. Riddle W. Misleading: The clinical implications of misplaced ECG leads. *JEMS.* 2008;33(9):56–62.
13. Kernicki JG. Differentiating chest pain: Advanced assessment techniques. *Dimens Crit Care Nurs.* 1993;12(2):66–76.
14. Tierney WM, Fitzgerald J, McHenry R, et al. Physicians' estimates of the probability of myocardial infarction in emergency room patients with chest pain. *Med Decis Making.* 1986;6:12–17.
15. Rouan GW, Lee TH, Cook EF, et al. Clinical characteristics and outcome of acute myocardial infarction in patients with initially normal or nonspecific electrocardiograms (a report from the Multicenter Chest Pain Study). *Am J Cardiol.* 1989;64:1087–1092.
16. O'Gara PT, Kushner FG, Ascheim DD, et al. 2013 ACCF/AHA guideline for the management of ST-elevation myocardial infarction: A report of the American College of Cardiology Foundation/American Heart Association Task Force on Practice Guidelines. *J Am Coll Cardiol.* 2013;61(4):e78–e140.
17. Antman EM, Anbe DT, Armstrong PW, et al. ACC/AHA guidelines for the management of patients with ST-elevation myocardial infarction: a report of the American College of Cardiology/American

Heart Association Task Force on Practice Guidelines (Committee to Revise the 1999 Guidelines for the Management of Patients With Acute Myocardial Infarction). *J Am Coll Cardiol.* 2004;44:e1–e211.

18. Bradley EH, Nallamothu BK, Stern AF, et al. The door-to-balloon alliance for quality: Who joins national collaborative efforts and why? *Jt Comm J Qual Patient Saf.* 2009;35:93–99.
19. Bradley EH, Herrin J, Wang Y, et al. Door-to-drug and door-to-balloon times: Where can we improve? Time to reperfusion therapy in patients with ST-segment elevation myocardial infarction (STEMI). *Am Heart J.* 2006;151:1281–1287.
20. Fisch C. Clinical competence in electrocardiography. A statement for physicians from the ACP/ACC/AHA Task Force on Clinical Privileges in Cardiology. *J Am Coll Cardiol.* 1995;25:1465–1469.
21. Michelson EA, Brady WJ. Emergency physician interpretation of the ECG. *Acad Emerg Med.* 2002;9(4):317–319.
22. Bradley EH, Curry LA, Webster TR, et al. Achieving rapid door-to balloon times: How top hospitals improve complex clinical systems. *Circulation.* 2006;113:1079–1085.
23. Lipton JA, Broce M, Lucas D, et al. Comprehensive hospital care improvement strategies reduce time to treatment in ST-elevation acute myocardial infarction. *Crit Pathw Cardiol.* 2006;5:29–33.
24. O'Connor RE, Brady WJ, Brooks SC, et al. Part 10: Acute Coronary Syndromes. 2010 American Heart Association Guidelines for Cardiopulmonary Resuscitation and Emergency Cardiovascular Care. *Circulation.* 2010;122:S787–S817.
25. Fox KA, Eagle KA, Gore JM, et al. The Global Registry of Acute Coronary Events, 1999 to 2009—GRACE. *Heart.* 2010;96(14):1095–1101.
26. Roe MT, Parsons LS, Pollack CV, Jr., et al. Quality of care by classification of myocardial infarction: Treatment patterns for ST-segment elevation vs non-ST-segment elevation myocardial infarction. *Arch Intern Med.* 2005;165:1630–1636.
27. Wright RS, Anderson JL, Adams CD, et al. 2011 ACCF/AHA focused update of the guidelines for the management of patients with unstable angina/non-ST-elevation myocardial infarction (updating the 2007 guideline): A report of the American College of Cardiology Foundation/American Heart Association Task Force on Practice Guidelines. *Circulation.* 2011;123(18):2022–2060.
28. Brieger D, Eagle KA, Goodman SG, et al. Acute coronary syndromes without chest pain, an underdiagnosed and undertreated high-risk group: Insights from the Global Registry of Acute Coronary Events. *Chest.* 2004;126:461–469.
29. Peterson ED, Rose MT, Mulgund J, et al. Association between hospital process performance and outcomes among patients with acute coronary syndromes. *JAMA.* 2006;295:1912–1920.

30. Sebbane M, Lefebvre S, Kuster N, et al. Early rule out of acute myocardial infarction in ED patients: Value of combined high-sensitivity cardiac troponin T and ultrasensitive copeptin assays at admission. *Am J Emerg Med.* 2013;31(9):1302–1308.
31. Amsterdam EA, Kirk JD, Bluemke DA, et al. Testing of low-risk patients presenting to the emergency department with chest pain: A scientific statement from the American Heart Association. *Circulation.* 2010;122(17):1756–1776.
32. Than M, Herbert M, Flaws D, et al. What is an acceptable risk of major adverse cardiac event in chest pain patients soon after discharge from the Emergency Department? A clinical survey. *Int J Cardiol.* 2013;166(3):752–754.
33. Winchester DE, Stomp D, Shifrin RY, Jois P. Design and implementation of a stand-alone chest pain evaluation center within an academic emergency department. *Crit Pathw Cardiol.* 2012;11:123–127.
34. Lee TH, Juarez G, Cook EF, et al. Ruling out acute myocardial infarction. A prospective multicenter validation of a 12-hour strategy for patients at low risk. *N Engl J Med.* 1991;324:1239–1246.
35. Roberts RR, Zalenski RJ, Mensah EK, et al. Costs of an emergency department-based accelerated diagnostic protocol vs hospitalization in patients with chest pain: A randomized controlled trial. *JAMA.* 1997;278:1670–1676.

CHAPTER 6

Risk Stratification of the Acute Coronary Syndrome Patient

Ki Park, MD

CASE PRESENTATION

45-year-old female with history of hypertension, no known prior history of coronary disease and not on aspirin presents with one episode of angina within the preceding two days with exertion, relieved with sublingual nitroglycerin. Serial ECGs reveal no evidence of infarct/ischemia and initial cardiac biomarkers are minimally elevated. She remains chest pain-free throughout her hospitalization without evidence of congestive heart failure or arrhythmias and otherwise remained hemodynamically stable.

INTRODUCTION

Unstable angina (UA) and non-ST elevation myocardial infarction (NSTEMI) encompass a spectrum of clinical presentations which are differentiated by whether the extent of myocardial injury is sufficient for detection by cardiac biomarkers. Unlike patients presenting with ST elevation myocardial infarction (STEMI), patients with UA/NSTEMI

Acute Coronary Syndrome: Urgent and Follow-up Care © 2017
Joseph S. Alpert, Lynne T. Braun, Barbara J. Fletcher, Gerald Fletcher, Editors-in-Chief,
Cardiotext Publishing, ISBN: 978-1-935395-94-2

do not necessarily warrant urgent coronary angiography/revascularization; thus there is more individualized discretion in determining future course of therapy based on timing and available options. Although these patients are not always subject to the immediate urgency as patients presenting with a STEMI, there is adequate evidence that UA/NSTEMI portends a worse prognosis in the long term as compared to STEMI.[1–4] Although these were older studies performed in an era where the primary revascularization strategy required the use of thrombolytics, it stresses the importance of accurate evaluation and managing these patients in a timely fashion to improve outcomes. This is particularly true for NSTEMI as these patients have a higher likelihood of residual ischemia.[1,5] In the GUSTO-IIb study, the presence of residual ischemia was associated with at least a doubling of the mortality rate. Thus, it is of utmost importance to risk-stratify these patients to make an assessment of their likelihood of future adverse cardiovascular events including recurrent myocardial infarction (MI), death, and recurrent angina.

RISK ASSESSMENT

Risk stratification begins upon first evaluation of the patient and should include assessment of multiple points including characterization of symptoms, risk factors, and laboratory data, including biomarkers. However, this should not be a static process as signs/symptoms of ischemia and subjective data including biomarkers may change over time. Thus, repeated risk assessment may be necessary as new clinical/laboratory data becomes available. An important point related to this is an evaluation by ECG. It is important to recognize that some patients may only have transient evidence of ischemia and that an ECG obtained while the patient is having active symptoms can be a valuable assessment tool.

Evaluation of risk aids in guiding immediate therapy, in particular deciding on the timing of coronary angiography, or whether medical management (an ischemia-guided strategy) may be more appropriate initially compared with an invasive evaluation. However, risk stratification is also a powerful prognostic tool to aid in managing the patient's long-term risk beyond the initial event. Several risk factor scores have been studied and are used in clinical practice and include the GRACE, PURSUIT and, perhaps best known, TIMI risk scores.[6–8] These scores vary somewhat in their specific components but generally rely on elements of both clinical history and objective data (see **Table 6.1**). General risk factors for consideration include advanced age, presence of known coronary disease, severity/timing of symptoms, heart failure/Killip class, and ECG changes/arrhythmias. When patients present with symptoms consistent with UA/NSTEMI, basic characteristics of their presentation such as symptom onset, whether symptoms are characteristic of angina, ECG changes and biomarkers, are important to immediately evaluate upon presentation. Assessment of left ventricular (LV) function within the first 24 hours is ideal as this can also help guide therapy. If there is evidence of localized wall motion abnormalities, this may suggest a role for early coronary angiography and revascularization as appropriate. Other high risk features favoring an earlier

Table 6.1
Comparison of TIMI, GRACE, and PURSUIT Risk Scores

	Age (≥65)	CAD Risk Factors	ASA Use	Prior hx CAD	Severe Angina	ST Changes	Positive Cardiac Biomarkers	HF/Killip Class	Hemodynamics
TIMI	X	X	X	X	X	X	X		
PURSUIT*	X				X	X		X	X
GRACE**	X					X	X	X	X

Additional elements: *gender, **cardiac arrest, creatinine

invasive approach include signs of cardiogenic shock, severe heart failure, recurrent angina despite maximal medical therapy, and hemodynamic instability/mechanical complications of MI such as mitral regurgitation or ventricular septal defect or unstable ventricular arrhythmias. Patients presenting with these feature should be referred for urgent cardiac catheterization (see **Table 6.2**). For these reasons, it is also important for continued vigilance and close monitoring of these patients during the early period after their presentation. This will also help guide in making a decision about what level of care they should receive, whether it be an intensive care setting versus a standard cardiac unit.

If a patient does not present with high-risk features, then risk stratification can aid in determining who should receive early, but not urgent, invasive evaluation with coronary angiography within the first 24 hours versus early conservative therapy. Early intervention is recommend in patients with positive biomarkers, ST depression on ECG, high-risk noninvasive testing findings, percutaneous coronary intervention within the previous 6 months, prior coronary artery bypass grafting, recurrent angina at rest or with minimal exertion despite maximum anti-anginal therapy, EF <40%, and high risk GRACE or TIMI risk score.[9–11]

Beyond the initial presentation, risk stratification is also beneficial to determine risk of future adverse cardiovascular events. Use of risk stratification scores such as TIMI, GRACE,

Table 6.2 Factors Favoring Early Intervention in NSTEMI
Cardiogenic shock
Severe heart failure
Recurrent angina despite maximal medical therapy
Hemodynamic instability/mechanical complications of myocardial infarction
Unstable ventricular arrhythmias

and PURSUIT continue to provide prognostic data throughout both the hospital course as well as up to a year beyond discharge. Once the patient's symptoms are stable, risk stratification should be reassessed and performed just prior to discharge or after discharge in medically managed patients who are at low initial risk or for various reasons opted to not undergo an initial invasive approach. These strategies primarily consist of LV function assessment and myocardial perfusion imaging to evaluate for evidence of residual ischemia and, if present, the extent of ischemia. This is generally reserved for patients who did not undergo coronary angiography due to either patient preference or other contraindication to angiography or were only partially revascularized. The method of stress testing may either include exercise or chemical stress testing, although exercise provides additional insight regarding a patient's functional status. Exercise testing is safe in patients whose symptoms/ECG have been stable in the preceding 12–24 hours.[9,11] Our initial case presentation highlights a clinical scenario of a low-risk patient, with a TIMI risk score of 1, in whom further risk stratification with noninvasive imaging would be most appropriate.

SUMMARY

Although guidelines for the risk stratification of acute coronary syndrome (ACS) have advanced significantly in the past few decades, areas for continued study exist. Recent studies have suggested that inclusion of other risk factors including anemia, renal dysfunction (currently only included in GRACE), as well as other biomarkers such as c-reactive protein and B-type natriuretic peptide may improve prognostic accuracy in initial evaluation. Thus, risk stratification of patients with UA/NSTEMI will continue to be an evolving process as new therapies and diagnostic tools become available.

REFERENCES

1. Armstrong PW, Fu Y, Chang WC, et al. Acute coronary syndromes in the GUSTO-IIb trial: Prognostic insights and impact of recurrent ischemia. The GUSTO-IIb Investigators. *Circulation.* 1998;98(18):1860–1868.
2. Furman MI, Dauerman HL, Goldberg RJ, et al. Twenty-two-year (1975 to 1997) trends in the incidence, in-hospital and long-term case fatality rates from initial Q-wave and non-Q-wave myocardial infarction: a multi-hospital, community-wide perspective. *J Am Coll Cardiol.* 2001;37(6):1571–1580.
3. Haim M, Behar S, Boyko V, Hod H, Gottlieb S. The prognosis of a first Q-wave versus non-Q-wave myocardial infarction in the reperfusion era. *Am J Med.* 2000;108(5):381–386.
4. Hasdai D, Behar S, Wallentin L, et al. A prospective survey of the characteristics, treatments and outcomes of patients with acute coronary syndromes in Europe and the Mediterranean basin; the Euro Heart Survey of Acute Coronary Syndromes (Euro Heart Survey ACS). *Eur Heart J.* 2002;23(15):1190–1201.
5. Wang CH, Cherng WJ, Hua CC, Hung MJ. Prognostic value of dobutamine echocardiography in patients after Q-wave or non-Q-wave acute myocardial infarction. *Am J Cardiol.* 1998;82(1):38–42.
6. Antman EM, Cohen M, Bernink PJ, et al. The TIMI risk score for unstable angina/non-ST elevation MI: A method for prognostication and therapeutic decision making. *JAMA.* 2000;284(7):835–842.
7. Boersma E, Pieper KS, Steyerberg EW, et al. Predictors of outcome in patients with acute coronary syndromes without persistent ST-segment elevation. Results from an international trial of 9461 patients. The PURSUIT Investigators. *Circulation.* 2000;101(22):2557–2567.
8. Eagle KA, Lim MJ, Dabbous OH, et al. A validated prediction model for all forms of acute coronary syndrome: Estimating the risk of 6-month postdischarge death in an international registry. *JAMA.* 2004;291(22):2727–2733.
9. Anderson JL, Adams CD, Antman EM, et al. ACC/AHA 2007 guidelines for the management of patients with unstable angina/non-ST-Elevation myocardial infarction: A report of the American College of Cardiology/American Heart Association Task Force on Practice Guidelines (Writing Committee to Revise the 2002 Guidelines for the Management of Patients With Unstable Angina/Non-ST-Elevation Myocardial Infarction) developed in collaboration with the American College of Emergency Physicians, the Society for Cardiovascular Angiography and Interventions, and the Society of Thoracic Surgeons endorsed by the American Association of Cardiovascular and Pulmonary Rehabilitation and

the Society for Academic Emergency Medicine. *J Am Coll Cardiol.* 2007;50(7):e1–e157.

10. Eagle KA, Guyton RA, Davidoff R, et al. ACC/AHA 2004 guideline update for coronary artery bypass graft surgery: A report of the American College of Cardiology/American Heart Association Task Force on Practice Guidelines (Committee to Update the 1999 Guidelines for Coronary Artery Bypass Graft Surgery). *Circulation.* 2004;110(14):e340–e437.
11. Wright RS, Anderson JL, Adams CD, et al. 2011 ACCF/AHA focused update incorporated into the ACC/AHA 2007 Guidelines for the Management of Patients with Unstable Angina/Non-ST-Elevation Myocardial Infarction: A report of the American College of Cardiology Foundation/American Heart Association Task Force on Practice Guidelines developed in collaboration with the American Academy of Family Physicians, Society for Cardiovascular Angiography and Interventions, and the Society of Thoracic Surgeons. *J Am Coll Cardiol.* 2011;57(19):e215–e367.

CHAPTER 7

Pharmacologic Management of the Acute Coronary Syndrome Patient

Andre R. M. Paixao, MD, and
Dharam J. Kumbhani, MD, SM, MRCP

INTRODUCTION

Since the first clinical trials establishing the benefits of aspirin and streptokinase in the 1980s, the evidence-based treatment of acute coronary syndromes (ACSs) has greatly evolved.[1,2] Contemporary pharmacologic treatment of ACS focuses on reducing myocardial oxygen demand, achieving and maintaining coronary artery patency, as well as preventing adverse cardiac remodeling and potentially fatal ventricular arrhythmias. With this in mind medications can be divided into six broad categories.

1. Anti-ischemic agents
2. Antiplatelet agents
3. Anticoagulants
4. Thrombolytics
5. Statins
6. Renin-angiotensin-aldosterone system (RAAS) inhibitors

Specific drug indications will often differ according to ACS subset. Patients presenting with ST elevation myocardial infarction (STEMI) will almost invariably undergo immediate reperfusion

Acute Coronary Syndrome: Urgent and Follow-up Care © 2017
Joseph S. Alpert, Lynne T. Braun, Barbara J. Fletcher, Gerald Fletcher, Editors-in-Chief,
Cardiotext Publishing, ISBN: 978-1-935395-94-2

through primary percutaneous coronary intervention (PCI) or chemical thrombolysis, and patients with non-ST elevation ACS (NSTE-ACS) will often be managed medically prior to invasive or noninvasive risk stratification. This chapter will focus on well-established indications of currently approved and commonly used medications, and the recommendations listed here are in general agreement with the most recent American and European guidelines.[3–6] **Figure 7.1** contains a brief overview of pharmacologic treatment options stratified by initial presentation and treatment strategy. **Table 7.1** lists medications commonly used in the treatment of ACS with respective doses, documented clinical benefits, and safety warnings.

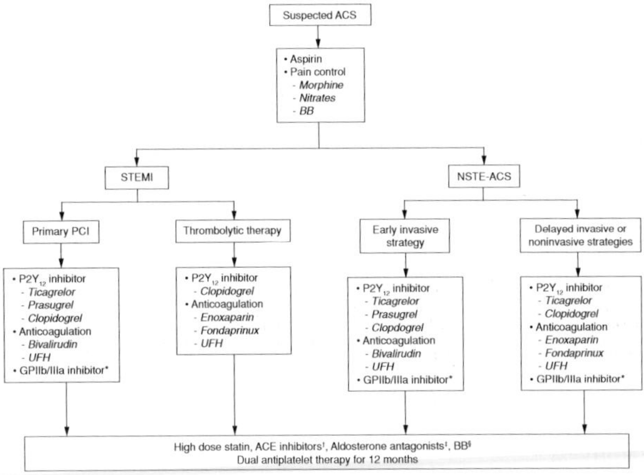

Figure 7.1

Overview of pharmacologic options for the treatment of acute coronary syndromes stratified by presentation and treatment strategy. ACS = acute coronary syndrome, BB = beta blocker, STEMI = ST elevation myocardial infarction, NSTE-ACS = non-ST elevation acute coronary syndrome, PCI = percutaneous coronary intervention, UFH = unfractionated heparin, GPIIb/IIIa = glycoprotein IIb/IIIa, ACE = ACE.

* In the setting of high thrombotic burden specially when using UFH. ** In high-risk patients with ongoing ischemia or when surgical revascularization is likely to be needed. † Benefits are better established in patients with large infarcts of depressed systolic function. ‡ In patients with depressed systolic function and heart failure or diabetes. § For 3 years in patients with myocardial infarction.

Table 7.1
Commonly Used Medication in the Treatment of Acute Coronary Syndromes

Drug Classes	Commonly Used Agents	Administration	Dose Adjustment	Clinical Benefit	Avoid/Caution
Nitrates	Nitroglycerin	SL: 0.3–0.6 mg every 5 min up to 3 doses; IV: 5–400 mcg/min	Not needed	- ↓ myocardial ischemia and BP - No impact on MI on CV death	- Suspected RV infarction - Hypotension - Recent use of PDE5 inhibitors
	Isosorbide dinitrate	SL: 2.5–5 mg every 5 min up to 3 doses	Not needed		
Beta blockers	Metoprolol	PO: 50–200 mg BID (100–400 mg daily if succinate)	Not needed	- ↓ myocardial ischemia, BP and HR - ↓ MI and CV death	- Signs of heart failure or shock - Profound bradycardia or heart block - Bronchospasm
	Atenolol	PO: 50–200 mg daily	Adjust in renal disease		
	Carvedilol	PO: 6.25–50 mg BID	Not needed		
	Esmolol	IV: 0.5 mg/kg bolus, 50–300 mcg/kg/min continuous infusion	Not needed		

(*Continued*)

Table 7.1
(Continued)

Drug Classes	Commonly Used Agents	Administration	Dose Adjustment	Clinical Benefit	Avoid/Caution
Calcium-channel blockers	Amlodipine	PO: 5–10 mg daily	Adjust in hepatic disease	- ↓ myocardial ischemia, BP, and HR - No impact on MI or CV death	- Hypotension - Bradycardia (non-dihydropiridine)
	Nicardipine	IV: 5–15 mg/hr	Monitor in renal and hepatic disease		
	Verapamil	PO: 80–160 mg TID (180–480 mg daily if extended release); IV: 2.5–5 mg over 2 min, second dose 5–10 mg after 15–30 min	Adjust in renal and hepatic disease		
	Diltiazem	PO: 30–80 mg TID (120–480 mg daily if extended release); IV: 0.25 mg/kg over 2 min, second dose 0.35 mg/kg after 15 min, 10–15 mg/hr continuous infusion	Not needed		
	Clevidipine	IV: 1–21 mg/hr	Not needed		

(*Continued*)

Table 7.1
(Continued)

Drug Classes	Commonly Used Agents	Administration	Dose Adjustment	Clinical Benefit	Avoid/Caution
Opioids	Morphine	IV: 2–8 mg every 5–15 min	Adjust in renal disease	- Pain relief - ↓ pulmonary congestion - No impact on MI or CV death	- Altered mental status - Hypotension - Bradycardia
Oral antiplatelets	Aspirin	PO: 162–325 mg initial dose, 75–162 mg daily maintenance dose	Not needed	- ↓ MI and CV death	- Hypersensitivity
	Clopidogrel	PO: 300–600 mg initial dose, 75 mg daily maintenance dose	Not needed	- ↓ MI and CV death when added to aspirin	- Excessive bleeding risk or anticipated need for urgent CABG
	Prasugrel	PO: 60 mg initial dose, 10 mg daily maintenance dose (5 mg if <60 kg)	Not needed	- ↓ MI but not CV death when compared with clopidogrel	- Excessive bleeding risk or anticipated need for urgent CABG - Age >75 years or prior stroke

(*Continued*)

Table 7.1
(Continued)

Drug Classes	Commonly Used Agents	Administration	Dose Adjustment	Clinical Benefit	Avoid/Caution
Oral antiplatelets	Ticagrelor	PO: 180 mg initial dose, 90 mg BID maintenance dose	Avoid in severe hepatic disease	- ↓ MI and CV death when compared with clopidogrel	- Excessive bleeding risk or anticipated need for urgent CABG
IV antiplatelets (GP IIb/IIIa inhibitors)	Abciximab	IV: 0.25 mg/kg bolus, 0.125 mcg/kg/min (max 10 mcg/min) continuous infusion	Not needed	- ↓ MI but not CV death when added to aspirin and standard anticoagulation	- Excessive bleeding risk
	Tirofiban	IV: 25 mcg/kg over 3 min, 0.15 mcg/kg/min continuous infusion	Adjust in renal disease		
	Eptifibatide	IV: 180 mcg/kg over 2 min, 2 mcg/kg/min continuous infusion	Adjust in renal disease		
Anticoagulants	Unfractionated heparin	IV: 60 units/kg bolus (max 4000 units), 12 units/kg/hr (max 1000 units/hr). Titrate to aPTT	Not needed	- ↓ MI when compared with placebo	- Excessive bleeding risk - History of HIT

(Continued)

Table 7.1
(Continued)

Drug Classes	Commonly Used Agents	Administration	Dose Adjustment	Clinical Benefit	Avoid/Caution
Anticoagulants	Enoxaparin	IV: 30 mg bolus SubQ: 1 mg/kg BID (max 100 mg)	Adjust if age >75 years or renal disease	- ↓ MI when compared with UFH in specific settings	- Excessive bleeding risk - Renal impairment - History of HIT
	Fondaparinux	IV: 2.5 mg bolus SubQ: 2.5 mg daily	Adjust in renal disease	- ↓ bleeding and CV death when compared with UFH and enoxaparin in specific settings	- Excessive bleeding risk - Renal impairment - Should not be used as sole anticoagulation in PCI
	Bivalirudin	IV: 0.75 mg/kg bolus, 1.75 mg/kg/hr continuous infusion	Adjust in renal disease	- ↓ bleeding and CV death when compared with UFH plus GP IIb/IIIa inhibitors	- Excessive bleeding risk

(Continued)

Table 7.1
(Continued)

Drug Classes	Commonly Used Agents	Administration	Dose Adjustment	Clinical Benefit	Avoid/Caution
Thrombolytics	Tenecteplase	IV: 30–50 mg weight based bolus	Not needed	- ↓ MI and CV death when primary PCI is not available	- Excessive bleeding risk - Carefully review general and specific contraindications
	Reteplase	IV: 10 units over 2 min, 10 units 30 min later	Not needed		
	Alteplase	IV: 15 mg bolus, 50 mg over 30 min, 35 mg over 1 hr	Adjust if <67 kg		
Statins	Atorvastatin	PO: 80 mg daily	Avoid in active liver disease	- ↓ MI, stroke, and CV death	- Caution with drug interactions - Monitor for myopathy and hepatic toxicity
	Rosuvastatin	PO: 20–40 mg daily	Adjust in renal disease and avoid in active liver disease		

(*Continued*)

Table 7.1
(Continued)

Drug Classes	Commonly Used Agents	Administration	Dose Adjustment	Clinical Benefit	Avoid/Caution
Angiotensin-converting enzyme inhibitors	Lisinopril	PO: 5–40 mg daily	Adjust in renal disease	- ↓ MI, stroke, and CV death in specific settings	- Hypotension or shock - Renal impairment or hyperkalemia - Bilateral renal artery stenosis - Angioedema
	Ramipril	PO: 2.5–20 mg daily	Adjust in renal disease		
	Enalapril	PO: 2.5–20 mg daily	Adjust in renal disease		
	Captopril	PO: 6.25–50 mg TID	Adjust in renal disease		
Angiotensin receptor blockers	Valsartan	PO: 20–160 mg BID	Adjust in renal and hepatic disease	- Noninferior to ACE inhibitors in ACS	- Hypotension or shock - Renal impairment or hyperkalemia - Bilateral renal artery stenosis

(*Continued*)

Table 7.1
(Continued)

Drug Classes	Commonly Used Agents	Administration	Dose Adjustment	Clinical Benefit	Avoid/Caution
Aldosterone antagonists	Spironolactone	PO: 12.5–50 mg daily	Adjust in renal disease	- ↓ MI and CV death in specific settings	- Renal impairment - Hyperkalemia
	Eplerenone	PO: 25–50 mg daily	Adjust in renal disease and avoid in severe liver disease		

PO = oral, SL = sublingual, IV = intravenous, BID = twice daily, TID = three times a day, min = minutes, hr = hours, BP = blood pressure, CV = cardiovascular, RV = right ventricle, PDE5 = phosphodiesterase type 5, HR = heart rate, MI = myocardial infarction, CABG = coronary artery bypass surgery, GP IIb/IIIa = glycoprotein IIb/IIa, UFH = unfractionated heparin, HIT = heparin-induced thrombocytopenia, SC = subcutaneous, PCI = percutaneous coronary intervention, ACE = angiotensin-converting enzyme, ARB = angiotensin receptor blocker.

ANTI-ISCHEMIC AGENTS

Nitrates

Intravenous (IV) or oral nitrates ameliorate ischemic symptoms by reducing left ventricular (LV) preload and slightly increasing coronary blood flow. They are currently used primarily for symptom relief and have not been shown to improve survival or attenuate myocardial injury.[7] Continuous nitroglycerin infusions are often used to control hypertension, ongoing ischemic symptoms, or pulmonary edema. All nitrates should be avoided in the setting of hypotension, marked bradycardia, suspected right ventricular (RV) infarction, and phosphodiesterase type 5 (PDE5) use within 48 hours of presentation. Nitrates are generally safe and administered to almost all patients in the prehospital setting.

Beta Blockers

Beta blockers (BBs) modulate catecholamine stimulation reducing myocardial oxygen demand by decreasing heart rate and contractility. Early studies have consistently reported reductions in recurrent myocardial infarction (MI) and cardiovascular death.[8] Anti-arrhythmic properties have also been well documented with significant reductions in ventricular tachycardia (VT) and ventricular fibrillation (VF).[8] In hemodynamically stable patients, BB should be initiated as early as possible. High doses of IV BB have fallen out of favor after they were noted to increase the risk of cardiogenic shock in a large randomized controlled trial (**Figure 7.2**).[9] For this same reason BB should be avoided in patients with signs of congestive heart failure (CHF) or at increased risk of cardiogenic shock. BB

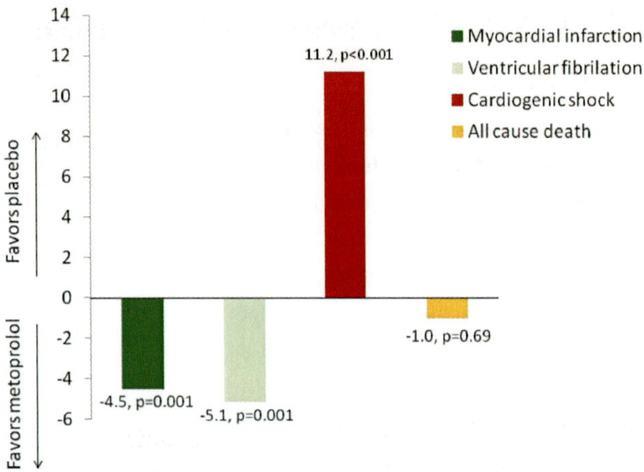

Figure 7.2

Absolute differences in outcomes per 1000 ACS patients treated with early high dose metoprolol.

should also be avoided in second- or third-degree heart block as well as active asthma. The duration of therapy has not been well established but most guidelines recommend continuing treatment for at least 3 years.

In the Clopidogrel and Metoprolol in Myocardial Infarction Trial (COMMIT), the early administration of high dose metoprolol was associated with fewer reinfarctions and less ventricular fibrillation but caused more cardiogenic shock with no significant effect on all-cause mortality.[9]

Calcium-Channel Blockers

Calcium-channel blockers (CCBs) reduce myocardial oxygen demand through negative inotropic and chronotropic effects (mainly nondihydropiridine agents) and result in systemic and coronary vasodilatation (mainly dihydropiridine agents). CCBs have not been shown to have an impact on survival or on the risk of reinfarction but are often useful to relieve ischemic symptoms and lower blood pressure especially when BB and nitrates are contraindicated. Nondihydropiridine agents (i.e., diltiazem and verapamil) should be avoided in the setting of marked bradycardia and CHF. Immediate release nifedipine should be avoided given the risk of hypotension and reflex tachycardia. All CCBs should be used with caution in patients with low blood pressure.

Analgesics

Morphine activates opioid receptors and is the analgesic of choice in patients with ACS. It reduces myocardial oxygen demand by reducing work of breathing and improving ventricular loading conditions. Its IV formulation usually provides prompt pain relief and often improves respiratory distress in patients with pulmonary edema. Caution is advised in patients with low blood pressure.

Nonsteroidal anti-inflammatory agents have been associated with increased mortality and should not be used in patients with ACS.

ANTIPLATELET AGENTS

Aspirin

Aspirin targets cyclo-oxygenase 1, inducing permanent platelet inhibition. Aspirin was one of the first agents shown to alter the natural history of ACS.[2] A loading dose of 162–325 mg should be given to all patients with suspected ACS and is often administered in the prehospital setting. A maintenance dose of 75–325 mg should be continued indefinitely. Low doses of aspirin are generally well tolerated long term and only modestly increase bleeding risks. Allergic reactions may occur and can be managed by desensitization or by switching to an alternative agent.

ADP Receptor Antagonists

These agents bind to the $P2Y_{12}$ receptor inhibiting adenosine diphosphate (ADP) mediated platelet activation. Ticlopidine was the first approved thienopyridine but has been mostly replaced by newer agents because of hematologic side effects. Thienopyridines such as clopidogrel and prasugrel, or the ADP receptor blocker ticagrelor, in conjunction with aspirin, will almost invariably be used in all patients with suspected ACS except for those with prohibitive bleeding risk or when urgent coronary artery bypass surgery (CABG) is likely to be the treatment of choice. Dual antiplatelet therapy should be continued for 12 months in all patients with true ACS irrespective of revascularization strategy. Interruption of dual antiplatelet therapy should be avoided for at least one month in medically managed patients or in those treated with bare metal stents and at least 12 months in those treated with drug eluting stents.

Clopidogrel

Clopidogrel continues to be the most widely used thienopyridine worldwide. It is a pro-drug, and is converted to its active metabolite, a carboxylic acid derivative, SR 26334, in the liver. In the CURE and COMMIT trials, it was shown to reduce the incidence of major adverse cardiac events (MACEs) in STEMI and NSTE-ACS irrespective of management strategy (invasive or noninvasive).[10,11] There has been debate about ideal dosing but a higher loading dose of 600 mg followed by 75 mg daily is generally preferred especially in patients undergoing primary PCI or an early invasive strategy. The prevalence of clopidogrel resistance has been reported to be as high as 30% but the extent of its clinical significance is still controversial. Genetic testing and platelet function monitoring have been proposed but clinical trial results have been disappointing and they are currently not recommended for routine use.[12–14] Compared with aspirin alone, the addition of clopidogrel increases bleeding risk but this seems to be outweighed by the reduction in ischemic events. Guidelines recommend that clopidogrel be stopped 5 days prior to surgical revascularization. In patients who are intolerant to aspirin, clopidogrel 300 mg as a bolus followed by 75 mg daily indefinitely is the preferred antiplatelet strategy for monotherapy.

Prasugrel

Similar to clopidogrel, prasugrel is a pro-drug but its conversion to active metabolite is subject to less individual variability, producing more potent and predictable platelet inhibition. In TRITON-TIMI 38, a 60 mg loading dose of prasugrel (after defining coronary anatomy but prior to PCI) followed by 10 mg daily was shown to reduce recurrent MI but not cardiovascular death when compared with clopidogrel in patients with STEMI and NSTE-ACS undergoing cardiac catheterization (**Figure 7.3**).[15] In NSTE-ACS patients treated with a

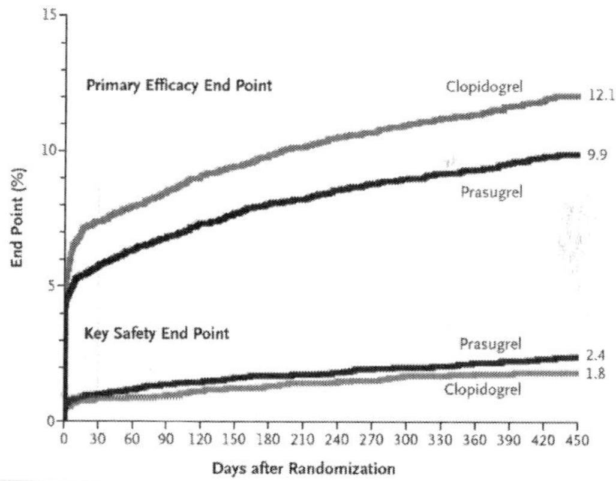

Figure 7.3

Kaplan-Meier estimates of the rates of key endpoints comparing prasugrel and clopidogrel in the treatment of ACS.

Primary efficacy endpoint = cardiovascular death, myocardial infarction, and stroke. Key safety endpoint = major bleeding not related to coronary bypass surgery.

(*Source:* Adapted from Wiviott et al.[15])

noninvasive strategy, no benefit was noted compared with clopidogrel.[16] Upstream use of prasugrel was also not beneficial compared with in-lab administration of prasugrel in NSTE-ACS patients.[17] Prasugrel was associated with an increased risk of bleeding compared with clopidogrel, and no net benefit was seen in the subgroup of patients over 75 years of age, weight <60 kg, or with a history of stroke. Most guidelines consider it a reasonable alternative in invasively managed patients outside that subgroup. The maintenance dose may be decreased to 5 mg daily in patients <60 kg. Prasugrel should be stopped 7 days prior to CABG.

Ticagrelor

Ticagrelor is a reversible allosteric inhibitor of the $P2Y_{12}$ receptor, but does not require biotransformation. Like prasugrel, it has a fast onset of action and results in very effective and predictable platelet inhibition. In the PLATO trial, ticagrelor administered as a 180 mg loading dose followed by 90 mg twice daily was shown to reduce MACE and cardiovascular death when compared with clopidogrel in patients with STEMI and NSTE-ACS undergoing invasive or noninvasive strategies (**Figure 7.4**).[18] Ticagrelor increased non-CABG bleeding, but a net clinical benefit persisted in all studied subgroups. Other side effects include dyspnea that is not associated with pulmonary edema, and ventricular pauses. These seem to be adenosine-mediated and generally do not require cessation of therapy. In patients undergoing CABG, the current recommendation is to withhold ticagrelor for 5 days.

Glycoprotein IIb/IIIa Receptor Inhibitors

The glycoprotein IIb/IIIa receptor mediates the final and common pathway of platelet aggregation, and is therefore an important target for antiplatelet agents. Glycoprotein IIb/IIIa

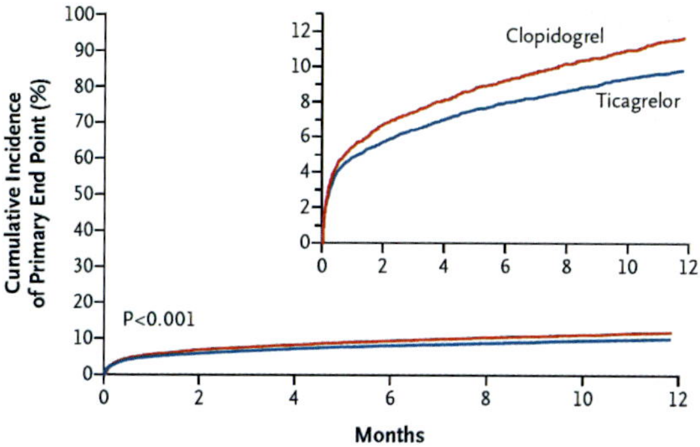

Figure 7.4

Kaplan-Meier estimates of time to first event comparing ticagrelor and clopidogrel in the treatment of ACS.

Primary end point = cardiovascular death, myocardial infarction, or stroke.

(*Source:* Adapted from Wallentin et al.[18])

receptor inhibitors are predominantly IV agents that produce very rapid platelet inhibition. Of the three agents available for clinical use, one is a large monoclonal antibody with prolonged pharmacologic effects (abciximab) and two are small molecules with much shorter duration of action (tirofiban and eptifibatide). These agents were initially tested before the wide spread use of thienopyridines and, when added to aspirin and unfractionated heparin (UFH), reduced recurrent ischemic events but not cardiovascular mortality.[19] Upstream use (i.e., prior to cardiac catheterization) has fallen out of favor[20,21] but they are still often used in the setting of large thrombus burden. Medically managed patients are also thought not to derive significant additional benefit when already treated with aspirin and a $P2Y_{12}$ inhibitor. Some have advocated its use in high-risk patients with ongoing evidence of ischemia when cardiac catheterization will be delayed by more than a few hours or when three-vessel coronary artery disease (CAD) is suspected and a $P2Y_{12}$ inhibitor will not be administered to avoid delaying surgical treatment. Eptifibatide was tested in the context of facilitated PCI (i.e., administered prior to angiography in patients with STEMI), but failed to show a benefit.[22] Important side effects include moderate to severe bleeding and thrombocytopenia. Marked reductions in platelet counts are more common with abciximab but also occur with the small molecule agents. Compared with heparin-induced thrombocytopenia (HIT), glycoprotein IIb/IIIa inhibitors cause a much faster and more severe drop in platelet count which is less often associated with thrombotic complications and can usually be managed by simply discontinuing the offending agent.

ANTICOAGULANTS

Short-term anticoagulation with IV or subcutaneous agents is generally recommended for all patients without prohibitive bleeding risk and continued until percutaneous or surgical revascularization is achieved. In the absence of successful revascularization and in patients treated with thrombolytics, anticoagulation should be continued for 48 hours or until discharge up to 8 days.

Unfractionated Heparin

UFH binds to antithrombin, augmenting inhibition of factors IIa and Xa. In the setting of ACS, it is administered intravenously and doses are titrated based on activated partial thromboplastin time (aPTT). Anticoagulant effects are short-lived and almost completely dissipated 4 hours after discontinuation of continuous infusion. It can also be promptly reversed with IV protamine. Early placebo controlled trials have demonstrated reductions in MACE, mainly by preventing recurrent MI. For invasively managed patients, an IV bolus is usually administered prior to cardiac catheterization, and a GPIIb/IIIa inhibitor can be added at the time of PCI. UFH may cause HIT, a condition associated with bleeding and thromboembolic events.

Low-Molecular-Weight Heparins

Low-molecular-weight heparins inhibit factor IIa and Xa without binding to antithrombin. They are well absorbed subcutaneously and have more predictable anticoagulant effect so that laboratory monitoring is generally not necessary. Anti-Xa levels can be assayed if clinically indicated. Enoxaparin has been well-studied in ACS. When compared with UFH in patients with NSTE-ACS, enoxaparin's noninferiority has been well established and, in patients treated with anticoagulation for at least 48 hours prior to PCI, it may be more efficacious in preventing death and MI. Enoxaparin is usually administered subcutaneously but can also be initially given intravenously, especially in patients undergoing PCI in whom it is being utilized as the sole anticoagulant. Doses should be adjusted in the setting of renal impairment and it should be avoided in those with more severe kidney disease. The incidence of HIT seems to be considerably lower when compared with UFH but bleeding risk may be slightly higher. Enoxaparin is generally not used in STEMI but is a reasonable option in medically managed patients with NSTE-ACS or when PCI is expected to be delayed by more than 48 hours.

Fondaparinux

Fondaparinux is a synthetic indirect factor Xa inhibitor with predictable anticoagulant effect and 100% bioavailability when given subcutaneously. In NSTE-ACS, when compared with enoxaparin, fondaparinux reduced the risk of bleeding as well as death or MI at 30 days, at the cost of higher incidence of catheter thrombosis in patients undergoing PCI.[23] When compared with UFH in patients with STEMI, a large randomized controlled trial yielded similar results, though no benefit was seen in the subgroup of patients undergoing primary PCI.[24] Fondaparinux should not be used in patients with severe renal impairment. No definitive cases of fondaparinux-induced HIT have been reported. Fondaparinux is a reasonable option in medically managed patients but is not recommended as sole anticoagulation in patients undergoing PCI.

Direct Thrombin Inhibitors

Several direct thrombin inhibitors have been tested in ACS but bivalirudin is the only agent endorsed by major guidelines. Bivalirudin provides fast and reliable anticoagulation with the theoretical benefit of inhibiting clot-bound thrombin and facilitating lysis of older thrombi. In HORIZONS-AMI, bivalirudin was compared with UFH plus GP IIb/IIIa inhibitors in STEMI patients resulting in lower risk of bleeding and better long-term survival, at the cost of a higher risk of early stent thrombosis. This thrombotic risk did not appear to be mitigated by upstream administration of bivalirudin and the use of more potent $P2Y_{12}$ inhibitors.[25] In patients with NSTE-ACS planned for an invasive strategy, two clinical trials yielded similar results though a survival benefit was not seen.[26,27] Few studies have compared bivalirudin with UFH without GP IIb/IIIa inhibitor. A recent randomized controlled trial inclusive of STEMI patients showed that UFH was associated with lower rates of ischemic events without increased bleeding risk.[28] The choice between UFH and bivalirudin remains somewhat controversial. Bivalirudin is currently not indicated for the treatment of medically treated patients with NSTE-ACS. Direct thrombin inhibitors are not associated with HIT, and conversion to bivalirudin in patients who have already received UFH seems to be safe.

Vitamin K Antagonists

Vitamin K antagonists (VKA) had once been a component of ACS management and secondary prevention, either in lieu of or in conjunction with aspirin, but in the reperfusion/dual antiplatelet era, these agents are limited to patients with a separate indication for anticoagulation (i.e., atrial fibrillation (AF), prosthetic heart valves, or venous thromboembolism). In the setting of LV thrombus or in patients with large anterior MI with depressed LV ejection fraction (LVEF) and apical akinesis, anticoagulation with a VKA for 3–6 months is usually recommended. The need for frequent laboratory monitoring and increase in bleeding risk are warfarin's major limitations.

Novel Oral Anticoagulants

These are oral agents, and do not require frequent laboratory monitoring.

Direct Factor Xa Inhibitors

Rivaroxaban and apixaban are the oral direct factor Xa inhibitors currently approved in the United States. They are approved for the treatment of venous thromboembolism and the prevention of thromboembolic events in patients with AF. In ATLAS ACS 2-TMI 51, rivaroxaban in reduced doses (2.5 and 5 mg daily) reduced the incidence of cardiovascular death, MI, or stroke in patients with ACS.[29] The reduction in ischemic events came at the cost of higher bleeding risks (including higher risk of intracranial bleeding), but a possible survival benefit was observed in the 2.5 mg daily rivaroxaban group. Rivaroxaban is not currently approved for use in ACS in the United States. Apixaban has also been approved for the prevention of thromboembolic events in patients with AF but not for the treatment of ACS. In the APPRAISE-2 trial, apixaban was tested in patients with recent ACS but the study was stopped prematurely because of an increased bleeding risk and the absence of significant reduction in ischemic events.[30]

Direct Thrombin Inhibitors

Dabigatran is the only oral direct thrombin inhibitor currently available for clinical use and has been approved for thromboembolism prevention in patients with AF. Dabigatran was tested in a small study of patients with recent ACS where it produced a dose dependent increase in bleeding[31] but has not been so far tested in a large trial of ACS patients. Pooled data from randomized studies of dabigatran show a possible increase in the risk of MI, which may be problematic in the setting of ACS.[32]

THROMBOLYTICS

Prior to the advent of primary angioplasty, IV thrombolytics were the treatment of choice for patients presenting with STEMI within 12 hours of symptoms onset. Since primary PCI has been shown to result in better vessel patency and lower mortality, chemical thrombolysis has been reserved for instances where PCI cannot be performed within 2 hours of medical contact.[33] In the narrow time window of 1–2 hours after symptoms onset, either strategy may be appropriate. Streptokinase was the first agent to gain FDA approval but is no longer available in the United States. Tenecteplase (TNK), reteplase (rPA), and alteplase (tPA) are currently marketed and seem to be equally efficacious. Careful review of general and specific contraindications must precede the administration of any of these agents.

LIPID LOWERING MEDICATIONS

Statins lower low-density lipoprotein (LDL) cholesterol by inhibiting 3-hydroxy-3-methylgluraryl-coenzyme A and are thought to have pleiotropic effects resulting in plaque stabilization. High-dose statins have been shown to reduce the

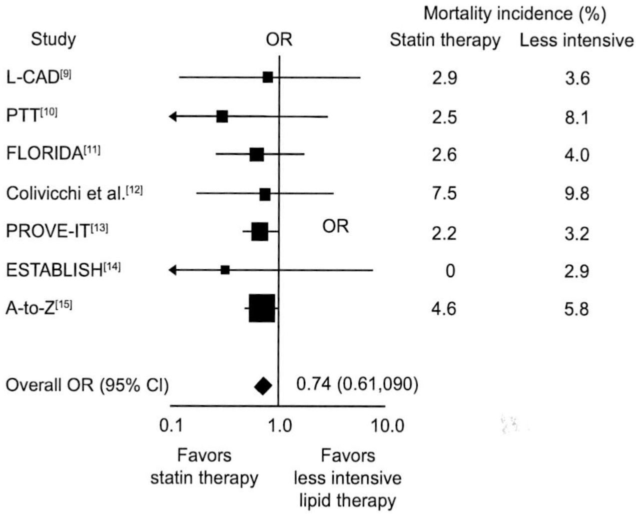

Figure 7.5

Odds ratio of all cause mortality for intensive versus less intensive statin therapy in acute coronary syndromes.

OR = odds ratio.

(*Source:* Adapted from Bavry et al.[35])

incidence of MACE in patients presenting with ACS and should be started irrespective of LDL levels (**Figure 7.5**).[34,35] There is also evidence that early administration of statins may be beneficial. In patients who are truly statin intolerant, lipid management should follow general secondary prevention recommendations.

RAAS INHIBITORS

RAAS inhibitors target different steps of this pathway resulting in reduced afterload and preventing cardiac remodeling. Angiotensin-converting enzyme (ACE) inhibitors reduce death and MI when administered early (within 24 hours) in patients with acute MI. This effect is more consistent in patients with STEMI and more pronounced in high-risk subgroups such as anterior MI, LVEF<40%, or CHF. ACE inhibitors are usually well tolerated but may cause profound hypotension, worsening renal function, marked hyperkalemia, angioedema, and cough. Angiotensin receptor blockers (ARBs) should be used in patients who are intolerant of ACE inhibitors. Cough and angioedema are not usual side effects of ARB. Both classes should be avoided in patients with hypotension, bilateral renal artery stenosis, or acute renal failure.

Aldosterone antagonists, more specifically eplerenone, have been shown to improve survival when started 3–14 days after an acute MI in patients with LVEF<40% and clinical heart failure or diabetes. Both eplerenone and spironolactone may cause profound hyperkalemia and should be avoided in patients with markedly elevated creatinine (>2.5 mg/dL in men and 2.0 mg/dL in women) or elevated potassium levels.

SPECIAL CONSIDERATIONS

Real-World Experience

ACS guidelines are populated by a plethora of randomized controlled studies. In real-world practice, there are frequent delays between the availability of new evidence and a commensurate change in clinical practice. At the other end though, these trials can sometimes be overly restrictive and often enroll less than 20% of screened patients. Study participants are closely monitored for adverse effects and frequently assessed by research nurses and coordinators. When medications and strategies are approved for use in real-world practice, they are often applied to a less restricted patient population (so called "indication creep") with less intensive monitoring and more variation in dosing and administration regimens.[36] For example, data from large national registries suggest that up to 40% of NSTE-ACS patients receive at least one inappropriate dose of antithrombotic agents and that bleeding risk increases with each degree of excess dose.[37] Older patients and those with renal disease are particularly vulnerable, with up to 20% receiving a contraindicated antithrombotic medication.[38] Large registries such as those maintained by the American College of Cardiology and the American Heart Association (AHA) now commonly collect and report data on practice patterns and real-world outcomes of ACS patients.

Need for "Triple Therapy"

Population trends along with the increasing use of invasive strategies for the management of ACS have resulted in the now frequently encountered scenario of older patients with multiple comorbidities and indications for both long-term systemic anticoagulation and dual antiplatelet therapy. Management of such patients with high risk of thromboembolic events (e.g., mechanical heart valves, AF, or recurrent venous thrombosis) and coronary stents is challenging. Multiple observational studies have reported markedly elevated bleeding rates associated with triple therapy with a 3-fold increase in risk compared with warfarin therapy alone.[39,40] In one relatively small randomized study, treatment with warfarin plus clopidogrel was associated with less bleeding compared with warfarin, clopidogrel, and aspirin without a detectable increase in ischemic events and with a possible survival benefit.[41] Since the novel oral anticoagulants are associated with less major bleeding and less intracranial hemorrhage, some have argued that the combination of these agents with aspirin and clopidogrel would be safer, but this was largely unproven until recently.[42] The recently published PIONEER AF-PCI trial revealed lower bleeding rates in patients treated with either rivaroxaban (15 mg daily) and a $P2Y_{12}$ inhibitor or rivaroxaban (2.5 mg twice daily) and dual antiplatelet therapy when compared with standard triple therapy.[43] Current guidelines still recommend that patients with recent ACS and an indication for anticoagulation should be treated with warfarin, aspirin, and clopidogrel and that the duration of "triple therapy" should be limited to the extent possible. The PIONEER AF-PCI trial may impact guidelines in the near future.

FUTURE DIRECTIONS

Clinical outcomes of patients with ACS have remarkably improved in recent years, but this is still one of the most active areas in clinical research. Data on two antiplatelet medications were recently published and deserve special mention. Cangrelor is an intravenously administered, fast acting $P2Y_{12}$ inhibitor with rapidly reversible antiplatelet effects. Initial studies yielded disappointing results, but a recent large randomized controlled trial reported reduction in MACE when compared with clopidogrel in patients undergoing elective or urgent PCI.[44] Though the magnitude of its benefit was modest and mostly limited to reducing intraprocedural stent thrombosis and periprocedural MI, cangrelor's favorable pharmacodynamics make it an attractive alternative in selected patients. Finally, vorapaxar is a protease-activated receptor blocker which inhibits thrombin-mediated platelet aggregation. In the TRACER study, vorapaxar reduced the incidence of cardiovascular death, MI, or stroke but with an unacceptably high bleeding risk (1.1% incidence of intracranial hemorrhage).[45] It was recently approved by the U.S. FDA in patients with ACS. A number of novel agents (antiplatelet agents, anticoagulants, and nonstatin lipid lowering agents) with different mechanisms of action are being investigated, and are in various stages of development. Several agents have already shown promising results in initial studies, and the future of ACS treatment seems to be bright as our understanding of vascular biology and interactions evolves.

REFERENCES

1. Effectiveness of intravenous thrombolytic treatment in acute myocardial infarction. Gruppo Italiano per lo Studio della Streptochinasi nell'Infarto Miocardico (GISSI). *Lancet.* 1986;1(8478):397–402.
2. Randomised trial of intravenous streptokinase, oral aspirin, both, or neither among 17,187 cases of suspected acute myocardial infarction: ISIS-2. ISIS-2 (Second International Study of Infarct Survival) Collaborative Group. *Lancet.* 1988;2(8607):349–360.
3. O'Gara PT, Kushner FG, Ascheim DD, et al. 2013 ACCF/AHA guideline for the management of ST-elevation myocardial infarction: A report of the American College of Cardiology Foundation/American Heart Association Task Force on Practice Guidelines. *Circulation.* 2013;127(4):e362–e425.
4. Jneid H, Anderson JL, Wright RS, et al. 2012 ACCF/AHA focused update of the guideline for the management of patients with unstable angina/Non-ST-elevation myocardial infarction (updating the 2007 guideline and replacing the 2011 focused update): A report of the American College of Cardiology Foundation/American Heart Association Task Force on practice guidelines. *Circulation.* 2012;126(7):875–910.
5. Steg PG, James SK, Atar D, et al. Task Force on the Management of ST Segment Elevation Acute Myocardial Infarction of the European Society of Cardiology: ESC Guidelines for the management of acute myocardial infarction in patients presenting with ST-segment elevation. *Eur Heart J.* 2012;33(20):2569–2619.
6. Hamm CW, Bassand JP, Agewall S, et al. ESC Guidelines for the management of acute coronary syndromes in patients presenting without persistent ST-segment elevation: The Task Force for the management of acute coronary syndromes (ACS) in patients presenting without persistent ST-segment elevation of the European Society of Cardiology (ESC). *Eur Heart J.* 2011;32(23):2999–3054.
7. GISSI-3: Effects of lisinopril and transdermal glyceryl trinitrate singly and together on 6-week mortality and ventricular function after acute myocardial infarction. Gruppo Italiano per lo Studio della Sopravvivenza nell'infarto Miocardico. *Lancet.* 1994;343(8906):1115–1122.
8. Freemantle N, Cleland J, Young P, Mason J, Harrison J. beta Blockade after myocardial infarction: Systematic review and meta regression analysis. *BMJ.* 1999;318(7200):1730–1737.
9. Chen ZM, Pan HC, Chen YP, et al. Early intravenous then oral metoprolol in 45,852 patients with acute myocardial infarction: Randomised placebo-controlled trial. *Lancet.* 2005;366(9497):1622–1632.
10. Yusuf S, Zhao F, Mehta SR, et al. Effects of clopidogrel in addition to aspirin in patients with acute coronary syndromes without ST-segment elevation. *N Engl J Med.* 2001;345(7):494–502.

11. Chen ZM, Jiang LX, Chen YP, et al. Addition of clopidogrel to aspirin in 45,852 patients with acute myocardial infarction: Randomised placebo-controlled trial. *Lancet.* 2005;366(9497):1607–1621.
12. Price MJ, Berger PB, Teirstein PS, et al. Standard- vs high-dose clopidogrel based on platelet function testing after percutaneous coronary intervention: The GRAVITAS randomized trial. *JAMA.* 2011;305(11):1097–1105.
13. Mega JL, Hochholzer W, Frelinger AL, III, et al. Dosing clopidogrel based on CYP2C19 genotype and the effect on platelet reactivity in patients with stable cardiovascular disease. *JAMA.* 2011;306(20):2221–2228.
14. Malinin A, Pokov A, Spergling M, et al. Monitoring platelet inhibition after clopidogrel with the VerifyNow-P2Y12(R) rapid analyzer: The VERIfy Thrombosis risk ASsessment (VERITAS) study. *Thromb Res.* 2007;119(3):277–284.
15. Wiviott SD, Braunwald E, McCabe CH, et al. Prasugrel versus clopidogrel in patients with acute coronary syndromes. *N Engl J Med.* 2007;357(20):2001–2015.
16. Roe MT, Armstrong PW, Fox KA, et al. Prasugrel versus clopidogrel for acute coronary syndromes without revascularization. *N Engl J Med.* 2012;367(14):1297–1309.
17. Montalescot G, Bolognese L, Dudek D, et al. Pretreatment with prasugrel in non-ST-segment elevation acute coronary syndromes. *N Engl J Med.* 2013;369(11):999–1010.
18. Wallentin L, Becker RC, Budaj A, et al. Ticagrelor versus clopidogrel in patients with acute coronary syndromes. *N Engl J Med.* 2009;361(11):1045–1057.
19. Tricoci P, Newby LK, Hasselblad V, et al. Upstream use of small-molecule glycoprotein iib/iiia inhibitors in patients with non-ST-segment elevation acute coronary syndromes: a systematic overview of randomized clinical trials. *Circ Cardiovasc Qual Outcomes.* 2011;4(4):448–458.
20. Giugliano RP, White JA, Bode C, et al. Early versus delayed, provisional eptifibatide in acute coronary syndromes. *N Engl J Med.* 2009;360(21):2176–2190.
21. Mehilli J, Kastrati A, Schulz S, et al. Abciximab in patients with acute ST-segment-elevation myocardial infarction undergoing primary percutaneous coronary intervention after clopidogrel loading: A randomized double-blind trial. *Circulation.* 2009;119(14):1933–1940.
22. Le May MR, Wells GA, Glover CA, et al. Primary percutaneous coronary angioplasty with and without eptifibatide in ST-segment elevation myocardial infarction: A safety and efficacy study of integrilin-facilitated versus primary percutaneous coronary intervention in ST-segment elevation myocardial infarction (ASSIST). *Circ Cardiovasc Interv.* 2009;2(4):330–338.

23. Yusuf S, Mehta SR, Chrolavicius S, et al. Comparison of fondaparinux and enoxaparin in acute coronary syndromes. *N Engl J Med.* 2006;354(14):1464–1476.
24. Yusuf S, Mehta SR, Chrolavicius S, et al. Effects of fondaparinux on mortality and reinfarction in patients with acute ST-segment elevation myocardial infarction: The OASIS-6 randomized trial. *JAMA.* 2006;295(13):1519–1530.
25. Steg PG, van't Hof A, Hamm CW, et al. Bivalirudin started during emergency transport for primary PCI. *N Engl J Med.* 2013;369(23):2207–2217.
26. Stone GW, McLaurin BT, Cox DA, et al. Bivalirudin for patients with acute coronary syndromes. *N Engl J Med.* 2006;355(21):2203–2216.
27. Kastrati A, Neumann FJ, Schulz S, et al. Abciximab and heparin versus bivalirudin for non-ST-elevation myocardial infarction. *N Engl J Med.* 2011;365(21):1980–1989.
28. Shahzad A, Kemp I, Mars C, et al. Unfractionated heparin versus bivalirudin in primary percutaneous coronary intervention (HEAT-PPCI): An open-label, single centre, randomised controlled trial. *Lancet.* 2014;384(9957):1849-58.
29. Mega JL, Braunwald E, Wiviott SD, et al. Rivaroxaban in patients with a recent acute coronary syndrome. *N Engl J Med.* 2012;366(1):9–19.
30. Alexander JH, Lopes RD, James S, et al. Apixaban with antiplatelet therapy after acute coronary syndrome. *N Engl J Med.* 2011;365(8):699–708.
31. Oldgren J, Budaj A, Granger CB, et al. Dabigatran vs. placebo in patients with acute coronary syndromes on dual antiplatelet therapy: A randomized, double-blind, phase II trial. *Eur Heart J.* 2011;32(22):2781–2789.
32. Uchino K, Hernandez AV. Dabigatran association with higher risk of acute coronary events: Meta-analysis of noninferiority randomized controlled trials. *Arch Intern Med.* 2012;172(5):397–402.
33. Keeley EC, Boura JA, Grines CL. Primary angioplasty versus intravenous thrombolytic therapy for acute myocardial infarction: A quantitative review of 23 randomised trials. *Lancet.* 2003;361(9351):13–20.
34. Cannon CP, Braunwald E, McCabe CH, et al. Intensive versus moderate lipid lowering with statins after acute coronary syndromes. *N Engl J Med.* 2004;350(15):1495–1504.
35. Bavry AA, Mood GR, Kumbhani DJ, et al. Long-term benefit of statin therapy initiated during hospitalization for an acute coronary syndrome: A systematic review of randomized trials. *Am J Cardiovasc Drugs.* 2007;7(2):135–141.
36. Kadakia MB, Desai NR, Alexander KP, et al. Use of anticoagulant agents and risk of bleeding among patients admitted with myocardial infarction: A report from the NCDR ACTION Registry—GWTG (National Cardiovascular Data Registry Acute Coronary Treatment

and Intervention Outcomes Network Registry—Get With the Guidelines). *JACC Cardiovasc Interv.* 2010;3(11):1166–1177.

37. Alexander KP, Chen AY, Roe MT, et al. Excess dosing of antiplatelet and antithrombin agents in the treatment of non-ST-segment elevation acute coronary syndromes. *JAMA.* 2005;294(24):3108–3116.

38. Tsai TT, Maddox TM, Roe MT, et al. Contraindicated medication use in dialysis patients undergoing percutaneous coronary intervention. *JAMA.* 2009;302(22):2458–2464.

39. Hansen ML, Sorensen R, Clausen MT, et al. Risk of bleeding with single, dual, or triple therapy with warfarin, aspirin, and clopidogrel in patients with atrial fibrillation. *Arch Intern Med.* 2010;170(16):1433–1441.

40. Lamberts M, Olesen JB, Ruwald MH, et al. Bleeding after initiation of multiple antithrombotic drugs, including triple therapy, in atrial fibrillation patients following myocardial infarction and coronary intervention: A nationwide cohort study. *Circulation.* 2012;126(10):1185–1193.

41. Dewilde WJ, Oirbans T, Verheugt FW, et al. Use of clopidogrel with or without aspirin in patients taking oral anticoagulant therapy and undergoing percutaneous coronary intervention: an open-label, randomised, controlled trial. *Lancet.* 2013;381(9872):1107–1115.

42. Moser M, Olivier CB, Bode C. Triple antithrombotic therapy in cardiac patients: More questions than answers. *Eur Heart J.* 2014;35(4):216–223.

43. Gibson CM, Mehran R, Bode C, et al. Prevention of bleeding in patients with atrial fibrillation undergoing PCI. *N Engl J Med.* 2016;375:2423–2434.

44. Bhatt DL, Stone GW, Mahaffey KW, et al. Effect of platelet inhibition with cangrelor during PCI on ischemic events. *N Engl J Med.* 2013;368(14):1303–1313.

45. Tricoci P, Huang Z, Held C, et al. Thrombin-receptor antagonist vorapaxar in acute coronary syndromes. *N Engl J Med.* 2012;366(1):20–33.

CHAPTER 8

Invasive Versus Conservative Treatment of Patients with Acute Coronary Syndrome

Calvin Choi, MD, MS, and Anthony A. Bavry, MD, MPH

DEFINITIONS OF ACUTE CORONARY SYNDROME AND MYOCARDIAL INFARCTION

Acute coronary syndrome (ACS) refers to constellation of symptoms due to myocardial ischemia and infarction, consisting of unstable angina (UA), non-ST elevation myocardial infarction (NSTEMI) and ST elevation myocardial infarction (STEMI). UA represents new onset or rest angina, changes in characteristics of chronic angina in frequency, intensity, or duration with or without ischemic changes on ECG such as ST segment depression or T-wave inversion and normal cardiac biomarkers. NSTEMI, on the other hand, represents signs and symptoms associated with UA associated with an elevation in cardiac biomarkers. STEMI represents an ACS with ST segment elevation in contiguous leads associated with abnormal cardiac biomarkers. Because cardiac biomarkers lag behind symptom onset, the initial assessment and treatment of the patient presenting with symptoms concerning for myocardial infarction (MI) should be the same. Early recognition and

Acute Coronary Syndrome: Urgent and Follow-up Care © 2017
Joseph S. Alpert, Lynne T. Braun, Barbara J. Fletcher, Gerald Fletcher, Editors-in-Chief,
Cardiotext Publishing, ISBN: 978-1-935395-94-2

prompt assessment and treatment of ACS are critical as there is a direct correlation between myocardial ischemic time and clinical outcome.

According to the European Society of Cardiology, the American College of Cardiology Foundation, the American Heart Association, and the World Heart Federation (ESC/ACCF/AHA/WHF) expert consensus document, MI refers to myocardial necrosis with a cardiac biomarker rise above the 99th percentile upper reference limit (URL), associated with symptoms suggestive of myocardial ischemia, new ischemic changes on ECG such as left bundle branch block (LBBB), pathologic Q waves, and ST/T wave abnormalities, angiographic evidence, or new wall motion abnormalities or a loss of myocardial viability on noninvasive imaging.[1]

Five different MI types are generally accepted. Type 1 represents MI which is typically associated with atherosclerotic coronary artery disease (CAD) and is due to intraluminal thrombus formation which may be caused by an acute spontaneous plaque rupture or a dissection. Type 2 represents MI due to supply and demand mismatch (e.g., profound hypotension, hypertension (HTN), bradycardia, tachycardia, anemia, respiratory failure, etc.). Type 3 represents death due to presumed ACS without cardiac biomarker assessment. Type 4a represents percutaneous coronary intervention (PCI) related MI (e.g., MI caused by procedure related embolization. Type 4a MI is defined by a cardiac biomarker rise above 5 times the 99th percentile URL for normal baseline or a cardiac biomarker rise of 20% along with symptoms suggestive of MI, new ischemic changes on ECG, angiographic evidence or new wall motion abnormalities or loss of myocardial viability on noninvasive imaging. Type 4b represents acute stent thrombosis with a cardiac biomarker rise above the 99th percentile URL. Type 5 represents coronary artery bypass grafting (CABG) related MI. Type 5 MI is defined by a cardiac biomarker rise above 10 times the 99th percentile URL along with a new pathologic Q waves or LBBB on ECG, angiographic evidence or new wall motion abnormalities or loss of myocardial viability on noninvasive imaging.[1]

RISK FACTORS

Lifestyle risk factors such as cigarette smoking, sedentary lifestyle, obesity, and diet high in glycemic index are associated with "Westernization" of developing countries and contribute to the increased global cardiovascular disease burden.[2] Noncoronary atherosclerotic disease, diabetes mellitus (DM), and chronic kidney disease are considered CAD equivalents. In addition, age, sex, HTN, a family history of premature CAD, dyslipidemia, mediastinum radiation, chronic inflammatory disease and metabolic syndrome are generally accepted risk factors for CAD.[3,4]

EVALUATION

The patients who present with symptoms concerning for an ACS will require urgent evaluation and triage. A focused interview and examination, risk profile assessment, cardiovascular, and pulmonary examination, along with laboratory values and noninvasive studies will guide management and treatment strategies. In particular, the ECG plays a critical role in guiding the initial treatment strategy. Because cardiac biomarker lags behind symptom onset, initial evaluation and treatment for an ACS should not depend on lab values; rather it should depend on a high clinical index of suspicion and the findings on ECG. Chest radiography, echocardiography, cardiac computed tomography angiogram, stress testing (exercise or pharmacologic), and/or cardiac catheterization can be used to guide evaluation and treatment strategies depending on the patient's clinical presentation and risk profile.

Irrespective of the initial evaluation and treatment strategies, all ACS patients require close observation, and frequent hemodynamic and clinical monitoring. The role of nursing is critical in this regard. Because ACS patients can deteriorate abruptly due to hemodynamic collapse or electrical instability, all ACS patients should be on a continuous monitor with frequent vital checks while a treatment strategy is formulated and carried out.

There is a direct correlation between prompt and efficient assessment, triage and treatment, and an optimal clinical outcome. Hence, a team approach to ACS management is encouraged. Emergency medical services, support staff, nurses, and physicians involved in an ACS management all play a vital role.

MANAGEMENT

Treatment Goals

Once an ACS diagnosis has been established, treatment goals should be determined based on a patient's risk profile, comorbidities, clinical status, overall prognosis, preferences, and ischemic burden, if known. In particular, bleeding risks and the need for noncardiac invasive procedures should be considered. Thereafter, a goal-directed therapy should be provided. First, supportive care should be provided if the patient is in extremis with hemodynamic or electrical instability. Second, symptom relief should be provided. Finally, the choice of a conservative or ischemia-guided versus an invasive strategy should be determined. A conservative strategy consists of aggressive pharmacotherapy while an invasive strategy refers to coronary angiography revascularization in appropriate patients with suitable risk profile, comorbidities, and anatomy. If a conservative or ischemia-guided strategy is selected as the mode of treatment then risk stratification with a noninvasive study prior to discharge from the index hospitalization is recommended.[5]

Conservative Strategy (Pharmacotherapy)

Antiplatelet Therapy and Anticoagulation

Atherosclerotic plaque rupture results in platelet adhesion, activation, and aggregation which cause flow limiting thrombus.[6] Furthermore, activated clotting factors contribute to thrombus formation. As such, antiplatelet therapy and anticoagulation are integral part of ACS pharmacotherapy. These topics are discussed in detail in Chapter 7: "Pharmacologic Management of the ACS Patients."

Fibrinolysis

The decision to administer thrombolytic therapy requires careful consideration. Namely, the potential benefits gained from intra-arterial thrombus resolution must be weighed against the risk of bleeding. A number of potential contraindications must be reviewed before thrombolytic therapy is administered.

For example, active internal hemorrhage; intracranial malignancy, arteriovenous malformation or aneurysm; and previous intracranial hemorrhage, aortic dissection, ischemic stroke or closed head trauma within 3 months and bleeding diathesis are all considered absolute contraindications. Relative contraindications include uncontrolled HTN (systolic blood pressure greater than 180 mmHg), ischemic stroke more than 3 months ago, prolonged or traumatic cardiopulmonary resuscitation (greater than 10 minutes), major surgery within 3 weeks, internal hemorrhage within 4 weeks, noncompressible vascular puncture, pregnancy, active peptic ulcer, and active anticoagulation.[7]

For UA and NSTEMI, thrombolytic therapy is contraindicated as the potential benefits do not justify the potential risk associated with the therapy.[8]

For patients with STEMI, thrombolytic therapy should be administered within 30 minutes of STEMI diagnosis. Thrombolytic therapy should be considered when patient transfer to a PCI center is expected to exceed 120 minutes.[9] The mortality benefit of the therapy is seen when the thrombolytic therapy is administered within 12 hours of symptom onset.[10] For elderly patients (age greater than 75 years old), the mortality benefits associated with thrombolytic therapy are less robust and should be used with caution. Thrombolytic therapy along with unfractionated heparin or LMWH, aspirin, and clopidogrel has been associated with improved outcome when compared to pharmacotherapy without clopidogrel.[11] Newer antiplatelet agents (prasugrel and ticagrelor) have not been studied with thrombolytic therapy. As such, ticagrelor or prasugrel should not be used in conjunction with thrombolytic therapy.

Streptokinase, alteplase (tPA), reteplase (rPA), and tenecteplase (TNK-tPA) are available agents. Streptokinase is the least expensive agent but it has inferior clinical efficacy compared to other agents and may result in hypersensitivity reactions (administer 1.5 million units over 60 minutes). Alteplase is administered as a bolus followed by infusion (15 mg bolus followed by 50 mg over 30 minutes then 35 mg over 1 hour for weight greater than 67 kg; 15 mg bolus followed by 0.75 mg per kg over 30 minutes then 0.5 mg per kg over 1 hour for weight less than or equal to 67 kg). Tenecteplase dosing is weight based and administered as a bolus (administer 30 mg for weight less than 60 kg, 35 mg for 60–69 kg, 40 mg for 70–79 kg, 45 mg for 80–89 kg, and 50 mg for weight greater than 90 kg). Reteplase is administered as two boluses (10 unit bolus followed by a repeat 10 unit dose in 30 minutes).[9]

Adjunctive Therapy

In theory, **supplemental oxygen** may improve hypoxemia (arterial oxygen saturation less than 90%) and increase oxygen supply to ischemic myocardium. However, this theory has not been proven in clinical trials. In fact, there is no definitive data to support the use of supplemental oxygen to improve mortality in the setting of ACS whether the patient is hypoxic or not.[12] The guideline-based use of supplemental oxygen is reserved for patients with a saturation less than 90%.

Furthermore, for the patients with chronic pulmonary obstructive disease, high dose supplemental oxygen may in fact suppress respiratory drive and result in hypercapneic respiratory failure. As such, routine supplemental oxygen therapy is inappropriate and selective use is encouraged. For significant hypoxemia in the setting of suspected ACS, underlying causes should be identified and treated; for example, pulmonary edema, pulmonary embolism, etc.

Nitroglycerin is an anti-angina agent available in various forms; for example, sublingual, intravenous (IV), patch, spray, etc. Nitroglycerin can improve myocardial perfusion by vasodilatation, resolving vasospasm, reducing wall tension and oxygen demand. However, because of its anti-hypertensive properties, nitroglycerin must be used with caution. For patients presenting with a suspected ACS, nitroglycerin should be avoided in the setting of hypotension (systolic blood pressure less than 90 mmHg), right ventricle infarct, severe aortic valve stenosis, bradycardia (heart rate less than 50 bpm), tachycardia (heart rate greater than 100 bpm) and use of a phosphodiesterase inhibitor for erectile dysfunction within 24 hours for sildenafil and 48 hours for tadalafil.[5]

Morphine has been an integral part of an ACS treatment protocol for generations. In fact, its use is so prevalent that "MONA," which stands for morphine, oxygen, nitroglycerin, and aspirin, has been taught in medical schools for decades. Morphine provides analgesia and relieves anxiety. However, its effect on ischemic myocardium is unclear. Recent, studies suggest that morphine may increase mortality in ACS cohort.[13] Consequently, routine morphine administration in the setting ACS should be avoided.

The benefits of **beta-blocker (BB) therapy** are well documented in chronic, stable systolic heart failure and the post

MI cohort. However, its role in the early phase of an ACS is unclear. In fact, studies suggest that IV BB administered in the early phase of an ACS may be harmful and increase cardiogenic shock and mortality.[14,15] A more prudent strategy may be to avoid IV BB in the early phase of an ACS and to defer oral BB therapy until the patient is clinically stable. Cardioselective BBs—metoprolol, atenolol are preferred over nonselective BBs.

Early intensive **statin therapy** has reduced adverse cardiovascular events in the setting of an ACS. In particular, atorvastatin 80 mg daily dosing has been studied in a number of large clinical trials and should be considered as the default agent.[16,17]

Invasive Strategy (Revascularization)

In the absence of contraindications, prohibitive comorbidities, or prognosis, the invasive strategy is preferred over the conservative strategy for ACS patients since a timely revascularization may improve mortality and clinical outcome.[18,19] This is true especially if a large ischemic burden exists. The decision to pursue the invasive strategy requires a careful and focused evaluation of the patients risk profile, comorbidities, prognosis, preferences, ischemic burden, and compliance with medical therapy. For the patients, with limited life expectancy or poor prognosis due to other comorbidities, the invasive strategy may not improve the overall clinical outcome.

A number of clinical trials have demonstrated benefits of the invasive over the conservative or ischemia-guided strategy in non-ST-segment elevation ACS. The Fast Revascularization during InStability in CAD (FRISC-II) trial compared the invasive versus the conservative strategy in non-ST-elevation ACS. In this study, 2457 patients were randomized to an invasive or conservative arm of the trial and followed for 5 years. The invasive strategy was defined as coronary angiography and revascularization (PCI or CABG) when appropriate within 7 days from admission. Five-year outcomes revealed the composite endpoint of death, MI, or both, favoring the invasive strategy (19.9% vs. 24.5%, $p = 0.009$). The benefits of the invasive strategy was seen in male gender, nonsmokers, and patients with two or more risk factors (age greater than 65, male gender, DM, previous MI, ST-segment depression, and elevated cardiac biomarker).[20]

In the Randomized Intervention Trial of Unstable Angina (RITA) trial, 1810 patients with non-ST-elevation ACS were randomized to an invasive (coronary angiography within 72 hours of randomization and revascularization when appropriate) or the conservative arm of the trial. At 4 months, the composite end point of death, MI, or refractory angina was superior in the invasive arm (9.6% vs. 14.5%, $p = 0.001$). The outcome was mainly driven by reduction in refractory angina in the invasive arm.[21]

In the comparison of early invasive and conservative strategies in patients with unstable coronary syndromes treated with the glycoprotein IIb/IIIa inhibitor tirofiban: treat angina with aggrastat and determine the cost of therapy with an invasive or conservative strategy (TACTICS-TIMI 18) trial, 2220 patients with UA and MI without ST-segment elevation were assigned to the invasive (coronary angiography within 4–48 hours after randomization and revascularization when appropriate) or conservative arm of the trial. At 6 months, the composite end point of death, nonfatal MI, or re-hospitalization for ACS was 15.9% for the invasive arm and 19.4% for the conservative arm ($p = 0.025$).[22]

The Invasive versus Conservative Treatment in Unstable coronary Syndromes I (ICTUS) trial is the most recent study to address the invasive versus conservative management strategies in NSTEMI patients. Investigators enrolled 1200 patients with NSTEMI who were assigned to an invasive (coronary angiography within 24–72 hours after randomization with revascularization when appropriate) or selective invasive arm of the trial. At 5 years, no difference was observed in the invasive and the selective invasive arms with respect to mortality or MI. However, the study results require careful interpretation. Unlike the FRISC-II, RITA, and TACTICS-TIMI 18 trials, the ICTUS trial had a significantly higher crossover to the invasive arm. In fact, patients in the invasive and the selectively invasive arms underwent revascularization at rates of 81% and 60% respectively. Due to significant crossover, ICTUS trial should be interpreted with the aforementioned detail in mind.[23]

Percutaneous Coronary Intervention

The decision to pursue a revascularization strategy entails several logistical concerns. The patient's potential bleeding diathesis, renal dysfunction, need for oral anticoagulation, need for a noncardiac surgery in the near future, ability to lie supine during PCI and compliance with medical therapy may sway treatment decisions during a PCI procedure. For example, the decision to implant a bare metal or a drug-eluting stent will largely depend on the aforementioned concerns. For the patients on a therapeutic oral anticoagulation, administration of reversal agents and a radial access may mitigate the bleeding risk associated with PCI. For morbidly obese patients, a radial access may also mitigate the potential bleeding risk associated with PCI.

For STEMI, current guidelines recommend a door-to-balloon time of 90 minutes or less as the goal for revascularization.[9] This is based on direct relationship between mortality and revascularization time; that is, the shorter the time from symptom onset to revascularization, the lower the mortality. For failed lytic therapy, a rescue PCI strategy may be performed but the potential risk for bleeding needs to be considered.[9]

For patients with UA/NSTEMI, guideline recommendations regarding an ideal time for coronary angiography are not well established. However, for patients with symptoms refractory to medical therapy, hemodynamic or electrical instability, urgent coronary angiography with an intention for revascularization is recommended.[5]

For the patients who present with an out-of-hospital cardiac arrest, an early invasive strategy is reasonable to consider, as recent data suggests that about one-fourth of the patients who present with an out-of-hospital cardiac arrest have an occult culprit lesion and a "silent" ECG without changes suggestive of ischemia, infarct, or injury.[24] In particular, for the patients who present with out-of-hospital cardiac arrest due to a ventricular arrhythmia, an early invasive strategy should be considered.

Coronary Artery Bypass Grafting

CABG may be pursued in the setting of an ACS if CAD is not suitable for PCI due to complex anatomy or the presence of a mechanical complication such as ischemic mitral valve regurgitation or ventricular septal defect.[25]

FOLLOW-UP CARE

At the time of discharge from the index hospitalization, ACS patients should receive sufficient education about ACS, the treatments they have received, medications, risk factor modification, prognosis, follow-up care, activity restrictions, and wound care when indicated. Elderly or disabled patients should be evaluated by physical and occupational therapists and social workers to determine their need for rehabilitation or support in the outpatient setting. For the patients without social support or financial means, the role of social workers is critical. Nutritional consultation is encouraged as many Americans are unfamiliar with a heart-healthy diet. Because ACS patients require a lifelong treatment, follow-up care and outpatient medications should be arranged prior to discharge from the index hospitalization to facilitate continuity of care.

When an ACS patient returns to clinic for a follow-up appointment, a careful history should be obtained to monitor the patient's progress and to assess the need for angina management. Inquiry regarding frequency, duration, and severity of angina will allow a provider to determine if the management strategy is adequate. If a conservative management has been pursued then risk factor modification (smoking cessation, heart healthy-diet, and HTN, dyslipidemia, and weight management) and optimization of anti-angina therapy are the priorities.

Furthermore, treatment related complications should be assessed. For example, anemia may be caused by antiplatelet therapy and procedure related blood loss; thrombocytopenia may be caused by antiplatelet agents such as glycoprotein IIb/IIIa inhibitors or heparin-induced thrombocytopenia (HIT); renal failure may be caused by contrast exposure. Mechanical complications from ACS are rare but can be severely detrimental—free wall rupture, ischemic ventricular septal defect or mitral valve regurgitation cannot be missed. Having a high index of suspicion, early detection, and treatment may offer the best chance at recovery and survival.

Focused examination should be performed to detect post-procedural complications if an invasive strategy was pursued. If PCI was performed then access sites should be examined thoroughly. Typically, PCI is performed through radial or femoral arteries and hemostasis is obtained by manual compression or a closure device. Closure devices are suture- or plug-based. Closure devices are not fail proof, nor are they safer than manual compression.[26,27] In fact, manual compression is generally accepted as the gold standard for hemostasis post-PCI. A careful examination is required to detect retroperitoneal bleeding, ischemia in the distal bed due to thromboembolism, or access site hematoma, dissection, arteriovenous fistula, pseudoaneurysm, or infection. Unexplained pain, hemodynamic, or electrical instability should prompt an urgent evaluation and further investigation with imaging studies when indicated; for example, ultrasound, CT, echocardiography, ECG, etc. If CABG was performed then sternal stability and wound healing should also be examined. Patients undergoing CABG often require the use of multiple invasive monitoring sites as well as cannulation for bypass pump and mediastinal tubes. As such, common access sites should be examined; for example, femoral artery/vein, radial artery, brachial artery, subclavian vein, and internal jugular vein.

Personalized Medicine

Personalized medicine is a new and promising field. Intense investigative effort has recently been allocated to this endeavor. In particular, antiplatelet therapy has been a topic of interest in cardiovascular medicine community. A number of studies have revealed that there is heterogeneity in the metabolism of antiplatelet agents in the overall population. Poor metabolizers may be at an increased risk for adverse cardiovascular events.[28] In theory, a tailored pharmacotherapy is attractive as it may improve clinical outcome at an individual level. Hence, the means to detect platelet reactivity has been studied extensively. However, adjustment of antiplatelet therapy based on platelet function or genetic testing has not resulted in improved clinical outcomes.[29–31] As such, until convincing data becomes available, pharmacotherapy should be tailored based on the patient's risk profile and clinical settings rather than on platelet function test or genetic profile.

Stent Thrombosis

Stent thrombosis is a rare post-PCI complication but the clinical implications are significant. Stent thrombosis is an acute event precipitated by thrombus formation within the stent due to vascular injury, incomplete stent expansion, delayed endothelialization, endothelial dysfunction, a hypersensitivity reaction or fibrin deposition.[32] The mortality rate associated with stent thrombosis has been reported to be as high as 45%. The incidence of stent thrombosis is about one to two percent and most events occur within the first month after PCI, irrespective of the stent type.[33] However, very late (beyond 1 year from the index procedure) stent thrombosis can occur as well. The most common causes for early (within the first month of the index procedure) stent thrombosis are premature discontinuation of dual antiplatelet therapy and mechanical complications such as incomplete stent expansion and vascular injury.[33]

Additionally, in the immediate post-PCI setting, close observation and monitoring are required as stent thrombosis can occur within hours after the index procedure. Because ACS patients are often sedated during a PCI, a high index of suspicion with prompt evaluation and treatment may mitigate detrimental sequelae.

Newer antiplatelet agents such as prasugrel and ticagrelor have been shown to have a lower incidence of stent thrombosis when compared with clopidogrel therapy in ACS patients who are treated with PCI.[28,34] As such, in the absence of contraindications and financial restrictions, newer antiplatelet agents should be considered as a default strategy in ACS patients who receive PCI.

Stent Restenosis

Stent restenosis is often confused with stent thrombosis. These two phenomena are distinct clinical entities and should not be confused. Stent restenosis has an insidious onset and is precipitated by vascular smooth muscle cell and intimal hyperplasia. As such, antiplatelet therapy has no role in the prevention of stent restenosis. The incidence of stent restenosis is about 4% to 8% with contemporary drug eluting stents. With bare metal stents, the incidence is about 10 to 15 percent.[35,36] Improved stent and polymer material and design, more potent anti-proliferative drugs, and refined delivery systems will likely reduce the incidence of stent restenosis even further.

Cardiac Rehabilitation

Cardiac rehabilitation is an under-utilized post-ACS therapy. After an ACS, patients often experience physical and emotional disability. In particular, for elderly patients, even a short hospitalization due to ACS can result in profound physical deconditioning. As such, a formal physical therapy evaluation along with a supervised exercise program can help facilitate a patient's ability to regain functional capacity, exercise tolerance, and physical independence.[37]

Finally, cardiac rehabilitation should also encompass risk factor modification, education, and vocational training. Even for patients with adequate social support, a personal illness can be an overwhelming experience. With reinforced education about their illness, and support from the heart team made up of the patient's cardiologist, primary care physician, nurses, physical therapists, and social workers, ACS patients can learn to live with and manage their illness, and to modify their risk factors. For the patients who require vocational training, cardiac rehabilitation can serve as a platform for reentry into the workforce. In turn, with comprehensive cardiac rehabilitation, the ACS patients can lead productive lives and learn to reduce their risk for future events.[37]

REFERENCES

1. Thygesen K, Alpert JS, Jaffe AS, et al. Third universal definition of myocardial infarction. *Circulation*. 2012;126:2020–2035.
2. *Global Status Report on Noncommunicable Diseases 2010*. Switzerland: World Health Organization, 2011. http://www.who.int/nmh/publications/ncd_report2010/en/. Accessed December 21, 2015.

3. Goff DC, Jr., Lloyd-Jones DM, Bennett G, et al. 2013 ACC/AHA guideline on the assessment of cardiovascular risk: A report of the American College of Cardiology/American Heart Association Task Force on Practice Guidelines. *Circulation.* 2014;129(25 Suppl 2):S49–S73.
4. Chung CP, Oeser A, Raggi P, et al. Increased coronary-artery atherosclerosis in rheumatoid arthritis: relationship to disease duration and cardiovascular risk factors. *Arthritis Rheum.* 2005;52:3045–3053.
5. Anderson JL, Adams CD, Antman EM, et al. ACC/AHA 2007 guidelines for the management of patients with unstable angina/non-ST-elevation myocardial infarction: A report of the American College of Cardiology/American Heart Association Task Force on Practice Guidelines (Writing Committee to Revise the 2002 Guidelines for the Management of Patients With Unstable Angina/Non-ST-Elevation Myocardial Infarction) developed in collaboration with the American College of Emergency Physicians, the Society for Cardiovascular Angiography and Interventions, and the Society of Thoracic Surgeons endorsed by the American Association of Cardiovascular and Pulmonary Rehabilitation and the Society for Academic Emergency Medicine. *J Am Coll Cardiol.* 2007; 50:e1–e157.
6. Davì G, Patrono C. Platelet activation and atherothrombosis. *N Engl J Med.* 2007;357:2482–2494.
7. Antman EM, Anbe DT, Armstrong PW, et al. ACC/AHA guidelines for the management of patients with ST-elevation myocardial infarction—executive summary: A report of the American College of Cardiology/American Heart Association Task Force on Practice Guidelines (Writing Committee to Revise the 1999 Guidelines for the Management of Patients with Acute Myocardial Infarction. *Circulation.* 2004;110:588–636.
8. Anderson HV. Intravenous thrombolysis in refractory unstable angina pectoris. *Lancet.* 1995;346:1113–1114.
9. O'Gara PT, Kushner FG, Ascheim DD, et al. 2013 ACCF/AHA guideline for the management of ST-elevation myocardial infarction: Executive summary: A report of the American College of Cardiology Foundation/American Heart Association Task Force on Practice Guidelines. *Circulation.* 2013;127:529–555.
10. Fibrinolytic Therapy Trialists' (FTT) Collaborative Group. Indications for fibrinolytic therapy in suspected acute myocardial infarction: Collaborative overview of early mortality and major morbidity results from all randomized trials of more than 1000 patients. *Lancet.* 1994;343:311–322.
11. Sabatine MS, Cannon CP, Gibson CM, et al. Addition of clopidogrel to aspirin and fibrinolytic therapy for myocardial infarction with ST-segment elevation. *N Engl J Med.* 2005;352:1179–1189.

12. Cabello JB, Burls A, Emparanza JI, Bayliss S, Quinn T. Oxygen therapy for acute myocardial infarction. *Cochrane Database Syst Rev.* 2013;8:CD007160.
13. Meine TJ, Roe MT, Chen AY, et al. Association of intravenous morphine use and outcomes in acute coronary syndromes: Results from the CRUSADE Quality Improvement Initiative. *Am Heart J.* 2005;149:1043–1049.
14. Kontos MC, Diercks DB, Ho PM, Wang TY, Chen AY, Roe MT. Treatment and outcomes in patients with myocardial infarction treated with acute ß-blocker therapy: Results from the American College of Cardiology's NCDR. *Am Heart J.* 2011;161:864–870.
15. Chen ZM, Pan HC, Chen YP, et al. Early intravenous then oral metoprolol in 45,852 patients with acute myocardial infarction: Randomized placebo-controlled trial. *Lancet.* 2005;366:1622–1632.
16. Cannon CP, Braunwald E, McCabe CH, et al. Intensive versus moderate lipid lowering with statins after acute coronary syndromes. *N Engl J Med.* 2004;350:1495–1504.
17. Schwartz GG, Olsson AG, Ezekowitz MD, et al. Effects of atorvastatin on early recurrent ischemic events in acute coronary syndromes: The MIRACL study: A randomized controlled trial. *JAMA.* 2001;285:1711–1718.
18. Milavetz JJ, Giebel DW, Christian TF, Schwartz RS, Holmes DR Jr, Gibbons RJ. Time to therapy and salvage in myocardial infarction. *J Am Coll Cardiol.* 1998;31:1246–1251.
19. Newby LK, Rutsch WR, Califf RM, et al. Time from symptom onset to treatment and outcomes after thrombolytic therapy. GUSTO-1 Investigators. *J Am Coll Cardiol.* 1996;27:1646–1655.
20. Lagerqvist B, Husted S, Kontny F, et al. 5-year outcomes in the FRISC-II randomised trial of an invasive versus a non-invasive strategy in non-ST-elevation acute coronary syndrome: A follow-up study. *Lancet.* 2006;368:998–1004.
21. Fox KA, Poole-Wilson PA, Henderson RA, et al. Interventional versus conservative treatment for patients with unstable angina or non-ST-elevation myocardial infarction: The British Heart Foundation RITA 3 randomised trial. Randomized Intervention Trial of Unstable Angina. *Lancet.* 2002;360:743–751.
22. Cannon CP, Weintraub WS, Demopoulos LA, et al. Comparison of early invasive and conservative strategies in patients with unstable coronary syndromes treated with the glycoprotein IIb/IIIa inhibitor tirofiban. *N Engl J Med.* 2001;344:1879–1887.
23. Damman P, Hirsch A, Windhausen F, et al. 5-year clinical outcomes in the ICTUS (Invasive versus Conservative Treatment in Unstable coronary Syndromes) trial: A randomized comparison of an early invasive versus selective invasive management in patients with

non-ST-segment elevation acute coronary syndrome. *J Am Coll Cardiol.* 2010;55:858–864.

24. Kern KB. Optimal treatment of patients surviving out-of-hospital cardiac arrest. *JACC Cardiovasc Interv.* 2012;5:597–605.
25. Hillis LD, Smith PK, Anderson JL, et al. 2011 ACCF/AHA Guideline for Coronary Artery Bypass Graft Surgery: A report of the American College of Cardiology Foundation/American Heart Association Task Force on Practice Guidelines. *Circulation.* 2011;124:e652–e735.
26. Nikolsky E, Mehran R, Halkin A, et al. Vascular complications associated with arteriotomy closure devices in patients undergoing percutaneous coronary procedures: A meta-analysis. *J Am Coll Cardiol.* 2004;44:1200–1209.
27. Koreny M, Riedmüller E, Nikfardjam M, et al. Arterial puncture closing devices compared with standard manual compression after cardiac catheterization: systematic review and meta-analysis. *JAMA.* 2004;291:350–357.
28. Wiviott SD, Braunwald E, McCabe CH, et al. Prasugrel versus clopidogrel in patients with acute coronary syndromes. *N Engl J Med.* 2007;357:2001–2015.
29. Price MJ, Berger PB, Teirstein PS, et al. Standard- vs. high-dose clopidogrel based on platelet function testing after percutaneous coronary intervention: The GRAVITAS randomized trial. *JAMA.* 2011;305:1097–1105.
30. Trenk D, Stone GW, Gawaz M, et al. A randomized trial of prasugrel versus clopidogrel in patients with high platelet reactivity on clopidogrel after elective percutaneous coronary intervention with implantation of drug-eluting stents: Results of the TRIGGER-PCI (Testing Platelet Reactivity In Patients Undergoing Elective Stent Placement on Clopidogrel to Guide Alternative Therapy With Prasugrel) study. *J Am Coll Cardiol.* 2012;59:2159–2164.
31. Collet JP, Cuisset T, Rangé G, et al. Bedside monitoring to adjust antiplatelet therapy for coronary stenting. *N Engl J Med.* 2012;367:2100–2109.
32. Farb A, Burke AP, Kolodgie FD, Virmani R. Pathological mechanisms of fatal late coronary stent thrombosis in humans. *Circulation.* 2003;108:1701–1706.
33. van Werkum JW, Heestermans AA, Zomer AC, et al. Predictors of coronary stent thrombosis: The Dutch Stent Thrombosis Registry. *J Am Coll Cardiol.* 2009;53:1399–1409.
34. Wallentin L, Becker RC, Budaj A, et al. Ticagrelor versus clopidogrel in patients with acute coronary syndromes. *N Engl J Med.* 2009;361:1045–1057.
35. Kandzari DE, Leon MB, Meredith I, Fajadet J, Wijns W, Mauri L. Final 5-year outcomes from the Endeavor zotarolimus-eluting stent clinical trial program: Comparison of safety and efficacy with

first-generation drug-eluting and bare-metal stents. *JACC Cardiovasc Interv.* 2013;6:504–512.

36. Hayes KR, Applegate RJ, Sacrinty MT, et al. Target lesion revascularization after bare-metal or drug-eluting stents: Clinical presentations and outcomes. *J Invasive Cardiol.* 2010;22:266–270.

37. Anderson L, Thompson DR, Oldridge N, et al. Exercise-based cardiac rehabilitation for coronary heart disease. *Cochrane Database of Systematic Reviews.* 2016; Issue 1. Art. No.: CD001800. DOI: 10.1002/14651858.CD001800.pub3

CHAPTER 9

Transitions of Care in Acute Coronary Syndromes

Eileen Handberg, PhD, ARNP-BC, R. David Anderson, MD, MS, and Kathy Berra, MSN, ANP-BC

INTRODUCTION

This book has provided the science underlying the pathophysiology of coronary artery disease (CAD) specifically related to acute coronary syndromes (ACSs), and guidelines for treating patients. The chapters have covered all phases of treatment with the goal of providing readers with the knowledge to improve care of patients with ACS. Achieving <90-minute door-to-balloon (D2B) times, preserving ejection fraction, and transitioning patients to home on guideline-recommended therapy are all goals of treatment. Once home, following a life-changing event, a key measure of the effectiveness of care is the level of success that patients have in resuming their lives armed with the knowledge and skills to implement risk reduction strategies known to reduce their future risk for cardiovascular events. This is a challenging task for patients, families, and providers. Data from the Centers for Medicare & Medicaid Services (CMS) indicate that while risk-standardized readmission rates and mortality rates for acute myocardial infarction (AMI) have decreased since 2010,[1] there is still an opportunity to improve transition to home as 1 in 5 AMI patients are readmitted within the first 30 days following hospital discharge.

Acute Coronary Syndrome: Urgent and Follow-up Care © 2017
Joseph S. Alpert, Lynne T. Braun, Barbara J. Fletcher, Gerald Fletcher, Editors-in-Chief,
Cardiotext Publishing, ISBN: 978-1-935395-94-2

The days of being cared for during hospitalization by your general practitioner, who has followed you since your birth, are long gone. The evolution in the delivery of medical care combined with mobility of society leads most patients to have a number of different healthcare providers over their lifespan. Patients will move, doctors will change practices, and insurance coverage will mandate changes in providers even for those who stay in the same location. As a result of these important changes, along with the development of the role of hospitalists and the increased utilization of specialists, the concept of continuity of care is becoming obsolete. In caring for patients with ACS, it becomes readily apparent that healthcare providers must work diligently to bring all the members of the healthcare team together in manner consistent with mobilizing an army, to provide the best quality of care throughout all of the phases of care. The effectiveness of this team is crucial to the success of the patient's experience during this health crisis. This chapter will discuss the challenges and opportunities facing the Care Team to improve the transition of the ACS patient through the many facets of our healthcare system. This will include identifying outpatient programs, guidelines, recommendations, and resources that can be utilized to improve quality of delivered care and improve both short- and long-term outcomes.

AWARENESS IN THE COMMUNITY—POPULATION-BASED APPROACHES

There are many "transitions of care" for a patient who develops chest pain. As illuminated in the previous chapters, this begins either with the first contact with the emergency medical system (EMS), a call or visit to the doctor's office, or after direct presentation to the emergency room (ER). ACS is an acute event that requires insight on the part of the patient or bystander that the symptoms they are experiencing require something more substantial than a "home remedy." Indecision is felt to be a key factor leading to delays in presentation,[2] and the literature is filled with studies designed to better understand the reasons for and ways to reduce these delays. Despite this, prehospital delay times have not changed significantly in the last 20 years.[3] With our in-depth knowledge regarding CAD and ACS, it may be possible to predict who is at highest risk to develop an ACS,[4] but unfortunately we cannot predict when an ACS will occur. Educating patients must be population-based with the hope of reaching those who are at highest risk and likely to develop ACS or those around them—that is, educating family, coworkers, and the general public about symptoms of ACS life-saving actions to take. While not the focus of this book, the first real opportunity to improve outcomes in ACS is developing and implementing a population-based strategy to educate the public about coronary heart disease, risk factors, symptoms suggestive of a myocardial infarction (MI) or ACS and the steps to take in the event symptoms develop.[5,6] The successful transition from someone with symptoms, to someone with symptoms who activates the healthcare system via EMS, contacts their healthcare provider, or goes straight to the ER in a timely manner plays a significant role in the effectiveness of ACS care and patient outcomes. The importance of these efforts were put in a scientific statement by the American Heart Association (AHA) in 2006,[2] reporting on the benefits of early treatment, factors related to patient delays in seeking timely treatment, and the limitations in our current approaches to decreasing these delays. Many organizations have taken an active role in creating community-based educational programs both traditional and, more recently, tapping into the power of social media. Mass media can efficiently facilitate reaching the public in a cost-effective manner.[7] These public health efforts support dissemination of education about the warning signs of a heart attack[8] as well as education for bystander cardiopulmonary resuscitation and use of automated external defibrillators. Equipping the public with skills to "act" when AMI or an episode of sudden cardiac death occurs will better assure quick action including alerting the EMS system. Once in the hands of the EMS, more complex transitions of care for patients with ACS begin.

PREHOSPITAL AND EMERGENCY ROOM CARE

As noted in Chapter 4, the EMS system has evolved into a very effective and efficient pathway for the care of person with ACS. Well-trained EMS personnel who work well with ER physicians, nurses, cardiologists, catheterization lab physicians, and other personnel can quickly transition ACS patients to effective treatment.[9–12] The transition of care from the point of EMS contact with symptoms of chest pain to the ER and to the cardiac catheterization laboratory has been streamlined with the D2B initiatives developed to improve outcomes.[13,14] The original goal of this intervention was to get patients from the ER door to having the balloon inflated in the occluded coronary artery within 90 minutes. Since its conception and implementation, this highly coordinated team-based approach has resulted in D2B times in many facilities of <60 minutes.[15,16] It also serves as a model of the importance of team-based care at its finest. In spite of these improvements, there still remains a risk-adjusted in-hospital mortality rate of 4.7% and an unadjusted 30-day mortality rate of 4.7%,[17] illustrating that in hospitals, even those with low D2B times, there is more work to be done. The transitions of care beyond the catheterization laboratory are where much opportunity resides.

Successful transition from symptom onset to therapeutic treatment is crucial to long-term outcome. Due to the necessary speed of the process, there is little time to do more than basic education of the patient, and available family members, about the disease process and the need for urgent intervention in that first 90 minutes. Ensuring all of the pertinent patient information and preferences for care are transmitted to members of the Care Team is extremely important as many patients may not have family members or caregivers readily available during this short window of care transition. When patients are in the middle of a life-changing, stressful, and often-painful event such as ACS, they may not be capable of fully understanding the importance of what has taken place. Several studies of care givers and patients have identified significant anxiety resulting from transitions of care. These include receiving conflicting information from multiple providers, lack of understanding as to the disease process and how to take care of themselves, and even a feeling of being left out of the decision making process as to the plan of care.[18–20] Often, the admitting nurse will serve as the provider who takes on the role of educating patients as to the plan of care as it evolves, serving as their advocate throughout the process, and making sure that family or appropriate friends/caregivers are contacted and, if available and appropriate, participate in decision making as care progresses.

IN-HOSPITAL CARE

The transition of the ACS patient from the ER to the catheterization laboratory and then to the inpatient unit offers unique challenges in providing continuity of care. The ACS patient has been taken to the cardiac catheterization laboratory and undergone coronary angiography, and may or may not have had a percutaneous coronary intervention (PCI) in the form of stent(s) placement, balloon angioplasty, or more complex procedures in the event of cardiogenic shock (intra-aortic balloon pump, Impella, etc.). These procedures are performed by an interventional cardiologist who often is a new provider to the patient. Depending on how hospital practices are set up, the patient may then be placed on a service staffed by the admitting interventional cardiologist and/or a partner in his/her practice, a hospitalist, or other medical service. In 2016, it is less likely the patient is cared for by his/her own primary care provider or a partner in that practice. Hospital coverage by groups, whether the cardiology or hospitalist practice, may lend itself to the patient seeing many practitioners who again are new to the patient, over the course of their 4–6-day hospital stay due to coverage schedules. With all of these changes in coverage providers, opportunities exist for breakdowns in communication leading to less-than-optimal care for the patient. Good communication across covering practitioners is crucial to ensure that quality care is delivered.

COMMUNICATION ACROSS PROVIDERS

The complexity of care and adverse outcomes associated with less-than-optimal care transitions has resulted in several professional societies examining and developing strategies to address this issue. The American College of Physicians, Society of Hospital Medicine, and other societies convened a working group that developed "The Transitions of Care Consensus Policy Statement." This important statement identified gaps in care and documentation where opportunities to improve care processes could make a significant difference in care transitions. In addition, the statement offered guiding principles to inform process improvement and some best practices for transition care documents.[21] While these issues relate mostly to inpatient-to-outpatient transitions, they also resonate for ACS care which by the nature of the treatment process has several inpatient transitions of care prior to hospital discharge.

Examples of Gaps in Care During Transitions

- In one cohort study of 400 patients, adverse events occurred in 1 in 5 patients and 66% were drug-related and could have been avoided.[22]
- Another study of 2644 patient discharges found that 40% of patients had pending test results at time of discharge and 10% required some action of which outpatient providers were unaware.[23]
- Direct communication between hospital and primary care physicians occurs infrequently (3%–20%).[24]
- The availability of the discharge summary at the first clinic visit after discharge is low (12%–34%) with some improvement after 4 weeks (51%–77%).[24]
- Discharge summaries, when available, often lack important information such as diagnostic test results, treatment, discharge medications, test results pending at discharge, or follow-up plans.[24]

Many of these communication breakdowns may result in adverse events and rehospitalization. CMS has instituted penalties for excessive readmissions of heart failure and post-MI patients which have led to hospitals and healthcare systems implementing new policies and processes to improve communication and improve transitions. The American Board of Internal Medicine (ABIM) Foundation in 2008 developed an initiative called "Stepping up to the Plate" (SUTTP) Alliance to develop standards to guide best practices. The SUTTP Alliance has developed five principals to frame efforts to achieve effective care transitions, and the Transitions of Care Consensus Conference[21] affirmed those principals and added four additional principals (**Table 9.1**).

Table 9.1 Five Principals for Effective Care Transitions
SUTTP Alliance
• Accountability
• Communication: clear and direct communication of treatment plans and follow-up expectations
• Timely feedback and feed-forward of information
• Involvement of the patient and family member, unless inappropriate, in all steps
• Respect of the hub of coordination of care
Transitions of Care Consensus Conference
• All patients and their families/caregivers should be able to identify their medical home or coordinating clinician (i.e., practice or practitioner).
• At every point along the transition, the patients and/or their families/caregivers need to know who is responsible for care to that point and who to contact and how.
• National standards should be established for transitions in care and should be adopted and implemented at the national and community level through public health institutions, national accreditation bodies, medical societies, medical institutions, etc. in order to improve patient outcomes and safety.
• For monitoring and improving transitions, standardized metrics related to these standards should be used in order to lead to continuous quality improvement and accountability.

Perhaps one of the most important components of the process is the Transition Record or Care Plan. This group developed a list of minimally acceptable data for this document, but also recommended several additional items that should be included in an ideal transition record (**Table 9.2**).

While some of these areas may not be necessary for an ACS patient, the complexity of interventions and need for long-term follow-up care make this a good model to be used by practitioners and healthcare systems to improve transitions of care.

Table 9.2 Transition Record or Care Plan
Minimal data to be included:
• Principal diagnosis and problem list
• Medication list (reconciliation) including over-the-counter medications/ herbals, allergies, and drug interactions
• Clear identification of the medical home/transferring coordinating physician/institution and the contact information
• Patient's cognitive status
• Test results/pending results
Ideal transition record to include the above and the following:
• Emergency plan and contact number and person
• Treatment and diagnostic plan
• Prognosis and goals of care
• Advanced directives, power of attorney, and consent
• Planned interventions, durable medical equipment, wound care, etc.
• Assessment of caregiver status

INPATIENT TRANSITIONS OF ACS PATIENTS

The transition to home for an ACS patient begins on admission to the inpatient unit from the catheterization lab. Once the patient is admitted, ongoing education continues and can be provided in a less urgent fashion. Ongoing education must include an understanding of the pathophysiology of ACS, the treatment(s) that were undertaken, and what further treatments will be recommended and prescribed based on guideline-recommended therapy and risk factor assessment. Given the pressure to reduce length of stay, with a mean hospital stay of 5.5 days nationally for ACS,[17] and the shifting nature of inpatient care, there is a greater likelihood for less-than-optimal patient education. While standardized order sets help to ensure that all of the important therapies are ordered, explaining the rationale for these therapies and assessing and then addressing important lifestyle changes requires strong communication. This should occur across all the members of the in-hospital team to ensure that patients receive all of the education they need and in the format that ensures the patient understands the information. Although order sets are standardized, patients are not. Assessment of each ACS patient and their life situation is necessary to ensure that the care provided meets the needs of the patient. Issues related to culture, literacy, socioeconomic limitations, and social support or lack thereof are all as important as the assessment of allergies and pertinent medial history. Patients are the focus of the team, but must be considered to be an integral part of the team.

A Scientific Statement from the AHA on transitions of care in heart failure outlines the prominent factors impeding transitions of care in chronic heart failure care,[25] many of which will exist for patients with ACS as well. The conceptual diagram was adapted to demonstrate the opportunities for team-based ACS care to reduce the impact of these impediments (**Figure 9.1**). With good integration of all the members of the healthcare team, physicians, nurse practitioners, physician assistants, pharmacists, nurses, cardiac rehabilitation specialists, social workers, and discharge planners, it is possible to leverage opportunities to support the patient during care. The areas are shown as overlapping because, depending on the staffing at the hospital/healthcare system, there may be several positions with similar areas of expertise to assist patients and families to overcome obstacles. For example, a pharmacist can assist with drug reconciliation, drug-drug interactions, as well as affordability. The social worker or discharge planner may also be aware of local pharmacies with lower costs, patient assistance programs for medical therapy, and may assist the patient with transportation issues to ensure appropriate

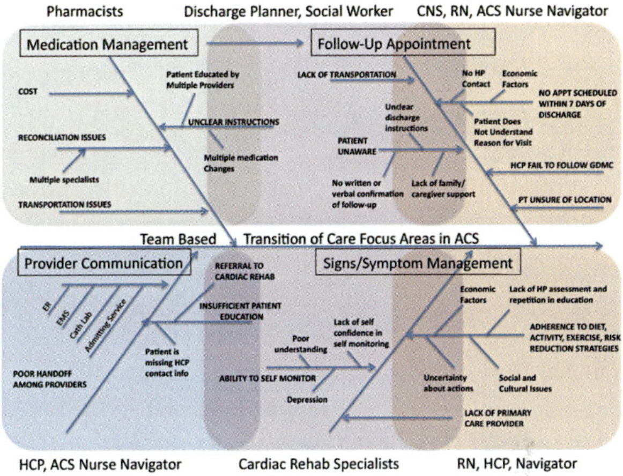

Figure 9.1

Areas of opportunities to improve team-based transitions of care in ACSs.

follow-up. All of these intersecting efforts, however, rely on strong communication between all the members of the team and most importantly with the patient and family.

Guideline-driven care is extremely important, but patients also require the financial, social, cultural, and emotional resources to be successful. Assessment of the patient and family status in all of these areas is an extremely important component of transition of care before discharge. For example, if an ACS patient has no prescription drug coverage, then prescribing ticagrelor as opposed to generic clopidogrel is probably futile, and may result in an early ACS event such as stent thrombosis if they are unable to afford to fill the prescription. The bedside nurse or the social worker should confirm potential financial constraints and communicate these findings to the pharmacist and healthcare provider. This will best ensure that the patient is prescribed the most effective and affordable treatment strategy which will result in improved compliance with recommended therapy and reduce hospitalizations and adverse coronary events.

With the advent of hospitalists managing inpatient care in many institutions, there are other challenges to maintaining the continuity of care. The patient really is the only consistent person in this entire interaction. To better align the care of ACS patients, the D2B team-based care mentality that has resulted in such extraordinary improvements in transitions from EMS to intervention needs to be mimicked. These approaches should be incorporated into an overall philosophy of EMS to Cardiac Rehabilitation framework where D2B transitions to a D2B-to-Cardiac-Rehab (D2B2CR) model to complete the evolution and transition of care that will optimize long-term outcomes. This requires extension of the systematized approach taken with D2B through to hospital discharge.

Part of the success of D2B is the clear role delineation of all the members of the "team," covering all aspects of the care. Successful D2B programs require strong, focused institutional leadership; extensive, organizational meetings to identify physician and nursing champions; identification of resources involved in the care of the patient; and clarifying provider roles. This coordination of care will result in patients receiving the care and education they need to be successful and safe following hospital discharge. Developing an ACS service from admission to discharge will create a more systematic approach and ensure that comprehensive care is consistently provided.

Many roles have evolved over the years to assist with transitions of care. It has always been the role of the bedside nurse to be a champion for the patient and take responsibility to coordinate or provide comprehensive discharge education. The increased utilization of pharmacists in the in-hospital setting, making them a part of team rounds, can improve the prescribing of appropriate therapy, decrease drug-drug interactions, and improve compliance with input regarding expense of medications, availability of combination therapy, and other factors.[26–28] While medical therapy is extremely important for ACS patients, further risk reduction with lifestyle changes cannot be undervalued. The complexities of successful lifestyle change for the patient and family are challenging but must be addressed.

In some facilities with strong cardiac rehabilitation programs, inpatient cardiac rehabilitation provides support for patient education regarding secondary risk-reduction strategies, specifically about activities of daily living, exercise, and lifestyle change. In some facilities, physical therapy takes on the acute intervention, and cardiac rehabilitation exists only in the outpatient setting. This transition to supportive post-discharge care is an important resource, but grossly underutilized as discussed in detail in Chapter 10.

ROLES SUPPORTING TRANSITIONS FOR ACS PATIENTS

ACS patients, because of the development of D2B and other initiatives, are transitioned quickly to lifesaving care. As this chapter has outlined, it is the management complexities beyond the catheterization lab that would benefit from a continuation of that type of structured, team-based model of care. A key to the achievement of optimal ACS care involves the identification of care champions as developed for the D2B programs, where institutional leadership combined with physician and nursing champions resulted in the most effective D2B programs.[29] Given the evolving complexities of care and need for additional support during and after discharge, whether to a rehab facility, use of a home health nurse/aid, or referral to outpatient cardiac rehab, numerous healthcare professionals in addition to nurses are necessary to facilitate these transitions. Due to the complexity of insurance, availability of resources (not all patients are local), and social support issues, new roles have evolved to take on this task. Depending on the institution, facilitating the transition to home has been led by a variety of positions to support the plan of care developed by the treating physician(s). This role has been part of the responsibility of the unit clerk in its simplest form to set up follow-up appointments and provide discharge paperwork for the patient, to more comprehensive management using case managers, social workers, or clinical nurse specialists. A new role has evolved to help with these complex transitions, often referred to as the Nurse Navigator. This role has evolved mostly from the cancer community and has been designed to facilitate patients' progress through the treatment process and healthcare organizational structures.[30] The Nurse Navigator role was started in 1990 at Harlem Hospital in New York to expedite diagnosis and treatment when facilitating access to care for patients with abnormal breast screening results.[31] The uptake of the Nurse Navigator in cardiovascular service lines is not yet widespread, but provides a comprehensive care model that can help ACS patients navigate complex healthcare systems during a life-changing healthcare event that has inextricably changed their lives.

RESOURCES

Resources for transitions of ACS care are found in many places. Information regarding guideline-recommended care for ST-elevation MI (STEMI) can be found on both the AHA website (www.heart.org) and the ACC website (www.acc.org) under "Guidelines." The American College of Cardiology has two programs that offer resources to assist with transitions for AMI patients. The Surviving MI Quality Initiative and Patient Navigator programs can be found at www.acc.org. Both of these quality initiatives offer assessments and toolkits to address a standard set of metrics. For the Surviving MI program there are eight metrics to measure program success:

1. Monitoring the hospital's AMI mortality data.
2. Hospital has evidence-based protocols and processes in place for AMI care, which continuously align with clinical guidelines and incorporate standard order sets.

3. Hospital has a champion team which includes a physician and nurse who work together to make decisions and are known as champions by the rest of the staff.
4. Hospital has an organizational culture which fosters and supports creative problem solving, such that:
   EMS providers review AMI cases at monthly meetings with physician/nurse champion, ED, and cardiac catheterization lab teams to identify lessons learned.
5. Hospital has access to cardiology expertise 24/7, ideally with an onsite cardiologist.
6. Hospital has specialized nurses dedicated to the cardiac catheterization laboratory and not shared with other units in the hospital.
8. Hospital should have a pharmacist actively involved in the management of AMI care.

The Patient Navigator Program combines registry data with toolkits to help hospitals and hospital systems implement processes to improve transitions of care with a focus on both heart failure and AMI. The metrics are shown below.

1. Compare Hospital using CMS Claims Data.
2. Thirty-day self-reported unadjusted mortality rate for HF and AMI patients.
3. Patient satisfaction is monitored quarterly.
4. Patient Quality of Life/Health Status.
5. Metrics from Action Registry "Get with the Guidelines Report."
6. Heart Failure Performance Measures (ACC/AHA).
7. HF and AMI patients are identified prior to discharge and risk of readmission is determined.
8. Medication reconciliation is performed accurately as appropriate for every patient *and* is documented in the medical record.
9. Follow-up visit or cardiac rehab referral (as appropriate) within 7 days is scheduled, documented in the medical

record, *and* patient is provided with documentation of the scheduled appointment (e.g., appointment card).

10. HF patient arrives at follow-up appointment within 7 days of discharge from hospital.
11. Discharge summary (including summary of hospitalization, updated medication list) available to follow-up clinician.
12. For HF and AMI patients, clinician discusses and provides documentation on the following:
    - Specific education on treatment regimen (self-care plan) and when to call their healthcare provider.
    - Documentation of all prescribed medications, instructions on when and how they should be taken, and about any changes to medications.
    - Community Resources for Healthcare.

These are just two programs that can be adapted and incorporated by hospitals or healthcare institutions to guide process improvement for ACS patient transitions of care.

SUMMARY

The ultimate success of ACS care for a patient includes the successful transition home with the ability to resume a productive life and to reduce the likelihood of further progression of their disease. As noted in the chapters of this book, medicine has made great strides in improving care for ACS patients with substantial reductions in mortality and morbidity over the last several decades. There continue to be opportunities to improve care through optimal use of guideline-directed therapy, improved communication, and utilization of the expertise of all the members of the healthcare team. This will ensure that the needs of the individual patient are assessed and practical solutions for care are developed to provide the patient and family the best opportunity for treatment success. This chapter has discussed the transitions an

ACS patient makes during their hospitalization to highlight where there is opportunity to improve care along the treatment path. CMS penalties for excess readmissions for AMI patients have provided a financial incentive for healthcare systems to more aggressively address these issues, and, with focused process improvement, ACS patients will benefit from these efforts.

REFERENCES

1. *Medicare Hospital Quality Chartbook 2014: Performance Report on Outcome Measures. Prepared by Yale New Haven Health Services Corporation Center for Outcomes Research and Evaluation for the Centers for Medicare and Medicaid Services 2014.* http://www.cms.gov/Medicare/Quality-Initiatives-Patient-Assessment-Instruments/HospitalQualityInits/Downloads/-Medicare-Hospital-Quality-Chartbook-2014.pdf. Accessed June 20, 2016.
2. Moser DK, Kimble LP, Alberts MJ, et al. Reducing delay in seeking treatment by patients with acute coronary syndrome and stroke: A scientific statement from the American Heart Association Council on Cardiovascular Nursing and Stroke Council. *Circulation.* 2006;114(2):168–182.
3. Nguyen HL, Gore JM, Saczynski JS, et al. Age and sex differences and 20-year trends (1986 to 2005) in prehospital delay in patients hospitalized with acute myocardial infarction. *Circ Cardiovasc Qual Outcomes.* 2010;3(6):590–598.
4. Goff DC, Jr., Lloyd-Jones DM, Bennett G, et al. 2013 ACC/AHA guideline on the assessment of cardiovascular risk: A report of the American College of Cardiology/American Heart Association Task Force on Practice Guidelines. *J Am Coll Cardiol.* 2014;63(25 Pt B):2935–2959.
5. Pearson TA, Bazzarre TL, Daniels SR, et al. American Heart Association guide for improving cardiovascular heath at the community level: A statement for public health practitioners, healthcare providers, and health policy makers from the American Heart Association Expert Panel on Population and Prevention Science. *Circulation.* 2003;107(4):645–651.
6. Pearson TA, Palaniappan LP, Artinian NT, et al. American Heart Association Guide for Improving Cardiovascular Heath at the Community Level, 2013 Update: A scientific statement for public health practitioners, healthcare providers, and health policy makers. *Circulation.* 2013;127(16):1730–1753.

7. Bray JE, Stub D, Ngu P, et al. Mass media campaigns' influence on prehospital behavior for acute coronary syndromes: An evaluation of the Australian Heart Foundation's Warning Signs campaign. *J Am Heart Assoc.* 2015;4(7):pii:e001927.
8. Garvey JL, MacLeod BA, Sopko G, et al. Pre-hospital 12-lead electrocardiography programs: A call for implementation by emergency medical services systems providing advanced life support—National Heart Attack Alert Program (NHAAP) Coordinating Committee; National Heart, Lung, and Blood Institute (NHLBI); National Institutes of Health. *J Am Coll Cardiol.* 2006;47(3):485–491.
9. Cone DC, Lee CH, VanGelder C. EMS activation of the cardiac catheterization laboratory is associated with process improvements in the care of myocardial infarction patients. *Prehosp Emerg Care.* 2013;17(3):293–298.
10. Johnston S, Brightwell R, Ziman M. Paramedics and prehosptial management of acute myocardial infarction: Diagnosis and reperfusion. *Emerg Med J.* 2006;23(5):331–334.
11. Pitta SR, Myers LA, Bjerke CM, et al. Using prehospital electrocardiograms to improve door-to-balloon time for transferred patients with ST-elevation myocardial infarction: A case of extreme performance. *Circ Cardiovasc Qual Outcomes.* 2010;3(1): 93–97.
12. Nestler DM, Noheria A, Haro LH, et al. Sustaining improvement in door-to-balloon time over 4 years: The Mayo Clinic ST-elevation myocardial infarction protocol. *Circ Cardiovasc Qual Outcomes.* 2009;2(5):508–513.
13. Krumholz HM, Bradley EH, Nallamothu BK, et al. A campaign to improve the timeliness of primary percutaneous coronary intervention: Door-to-balloon: An alliance for quality. *JACC Cardiovasc Interv.* 2008:1(1):97–104.
14. Jacobs AK, Antman E, Ellrodt G, et al. Recommendation to develop strategies to increase the number of ST-segment-elevation myocardial infarction patients with timely access to primary percutaneous coronary intervention. *Circulation.* 2006;113(17):2152–2163.
15. Krumholz HM, Herrin J, Miller LE, et al. Improvements in door-to-balloon time in the United States, 2005 to 2010. *Circulation.* 2011;124(9):1038–1045.
16. Menees DS, Peterson ED, Wang Y, et al. Door-to-balloon time and mortality among patients undergoing primary PCI. *N Engl J Med.* 2013;369(10):901–909.
17. LaMori JC, Shoheiber O, Dudash K, Crivera C, Mody SH. The economic impact of acute coronary syndrome on length of stay: An analysis using the Healthcare Cost and Utilization Project (HCUP) databases. *J Med Econ.* 2014;17(3):191–197.

18. Coleman EA, Smith JD, Franc JC, Eilertsen TB, Thiare JN, Kramer AM. Development and testing of a measure designed to assess the quality of care transitions. *Int J Integr Care*. 2002;2:e02.
19. vom Eigen KA, Walker JD, Edgman-Levitan S, Cleary PD, Delbanco TL. Carepartner experiences with hospital care. *Med Care*. 1999;37(1):33–38.
20. Coleman EA, Mahoney E, Parry C. Assessing the quality of preparation for posthospital care from the patient's perspective: The Care Transitions Measure. *Med Care*. 2005;43(3):246–255.
21. Snow V, Beck D, Budnitz T, et al. Transitions of Care Consensus Policy Statement: American College of Physicians, Society of General Internal Medicine, Society of Hospital Medicine, American Geriatrics Society, American College of Emergency Physicians, and Society of Academic Emergency Medicine. *J Hosp Med*. 2009;4(6):364–370.
22. Forster AJ, Murff HJ, Peterson JF, Gandhi TK, Bates DW. The incidence and severity of adverse events affecting patients after discharge from the hospital. *Ann Intern Med*. 2003;138(3):161–167.
23. Roy CL, Poon EG, Karson AS, et al. Patient safety concerns arising from test results that return after hospital discharge. *Ann Intern Med*. 2005;143(2):121–128.
24. Kripalani S, LeFevre F, Phillips CO, Williams MV, Basaviah P, Baker DW. Deficits in communication and information transfer between hospital-based and primary care physicians: Implications for patient safety and continuity of care. *JAMA*. 2007;297(8):831–841.
25. Albert NM, Barnason S, Deswal A, et al. Transitions of care in heart failure: A scientific statement from the American Heart Association. *Circ Heart Fail*. 2015;8(2):384–409.
26. Bradley EH, Curry LA, Spatz ES, et al. Hospital strategies for reducing risk-standardized mortality rates in acute myocardial infarction. *Ann Intern Med*. 2012;156(9):618–626.
27. Bond CA, Raehl CL. Clinical pharmacy services, pharmacy staffing, and hospital mortality rates. *Pharmacotherapy*. 2007;27(4):481–493.
28. Axtell SS, Ludwig E, Lopez–Candales A. Intervention to improve adherence to ACC/AHA recommended adjunctive medications for the management of patients with an acute myocardial infarction. *Clin Cardiol*. 2001;24(2):114–118.
29. Curry LA, Spatz E, Cherlin E, et al. What distinguishes top-performing hospitals in acute myocardial infarction rates? A qualitative study. *Ann Intern Med*. 2011;154(6):384–390.
30. Pruitt Z, Sportsman S. The presence and roles of nurse navigators in acute care hospitals. *J Nurs Adm*. 2013;43(11):592–596.
31. Pedersen A, Hack TF. Pilots of oncology health care: A concept analysis of the patient navigator role. *Oncol Nurs Forum*. 2010;37(1):55–60.

CHAPTER 10

The Role of Cardiac Rehabilitation After an Acute Coronary Syndrome

Ty J. Gluckman, MD, and Andrew M. Freeman, MD

INTRODUCTION

Each year in the United States, approximately 1.1 million individuals are diagnosed with an acute coronary syndrome (ACS).[1] This diagnosis includes the three related conditions of ST-segment elevation myocardial infarction (STEMI), non-ST-segment elevation myocardial infarction (NSTEMI), and unstable angina (UA). While recognized as distinct entities, these events represent a continuum resulting from coronary plaque erosion or rupture with subsequent complete or partial occlusion of the coronary artery with thrombus.[2]

Unequivocally, disproportionate attention is paid to these patients in their acute management. Important decisions revolve around whether STEMI patients should receive percutaneous or pharmacologic reperfusion or whether an early invasive or early conservative strategy is warranted for those with a non-ST-segment elevation ACS (NSTE-ACS). Even though first line medical therapies (e.g., ACE inhibitors or angiotensin receptor blockers, beta blockers [BBs], and statins), are frequently initiated, it is usually with an eye toward reducing near-term events.

Acute Coronary Syndrome: Urgent and Follow-up Care © 2017
Joseph S. Alpert, Lynne T. Braun, Barbara J. Fletcher, Gerald Fletcher, Editors-in-Chief,
Cardiotext Publishing, ISBN: 978-1-935395-94-2

Unfortunately, ACS patients remain at high risk for recurrent cardiovascular (CV) events well beyond this time frame.[3] The continued use of risk-reducing medications is paramount and accounts for nearly half of the reduction in coronary heart disease (CHD) mortality that has been observed over the last decade.[4] In addition, lifestyle interventions play an important role and include tobacco cessation, weight reduction through diet and exercise, and stress management. Behavioral health problems (i.e., depression) must also be addressed, as they can impact long-term compliance with risk-reducing interventions. In spite of the fact that most of the remaining decline in CHD mortality that has occurred over the last decade has been due to reductions in population-wide risk factors,[4] these nonpharmacologic interventions are usually not initiated with the same intensity.

Cardiac rehabilitation offers the advantage of addressing both aspects of CV risk reduction. While it is highly cost-effective, referral to and enrollment in dedicated programs is disappointingly poor.[5,6] Even though the reasons for this are likely numerous, limited reimbursement for preventive efforts likely plays a big role. Given the systemic underuse of cardiac rehabilitation, this chapter will provide readers with an understanding of 1) its core competencies (particularly for patients following an ACS), 2) its clinical benefits, and 3) the myths contributing to its underutilization.

WHAT IS CARDIAC REHABILITATION?

Cardiac rehabilitation is a comprehensive supervised program consisting of an initial medical evaluation followed by prescribed exercise, CV risk factor modification, and educational, counseling, and behavioral interventions.[7] It is a Class I, Level of Evidence (LOE) B recommended therapy following a STEMI[8] and an NSTE-ACS,[9] regardless of whether revascularization was performed.

Cardiac rehabilitation is traditionally divided into 4 phases. Phase 1 occurs during the initial acute inpatient hospitalization. Phase 2, which is the most familiar phase, occurs in the immediate outpatient period and usually lasts 12–18 weeks, with sessions occurring 2–3 times per week for a total of 36 sessions. It is the most monitored phase of rehabilitation. Phase 3 occurs immediately following the completion of phase 2 and is generally considered an intermediate phase where patients participate in the same types of exercise training and lifestyle change but are not as closely supervised. Finally, phase 4 is a transition to long-term maintenance of all of the healthful behaviors that were learned in the previous phases to achieve long-term CV risk reduction.

In 2007, the American Heart Association (AHA) and the American Association of Cardiovascular and Pulmonary Rehabilitation (AACVPR) published the core components of cardiac rehabilitation and secondary prevention programs (**Table 10.1**).[10] For each component, specific evaluation,

Table 10.1
Core Components of Cardiac Rehabilitation and Secondary Prevention Programs[10]

Core Components
1. Initial patient assessment
2. Nutritional counseling
3. Weight management
4. Blood pressure management
5. Lipid management
6. Diabetes management
7. Tobacco cessation
8. Psychosocial management
9. Physical activity counseling and exercise training

intervention, and expected outcome recommendations were made. These components were intended to assist staff in designing and developing programs, as well as to define standards for certification.

Initial Patient Assessment

Following an ACS, assessment of prognosis is an important step to manage the risk of future adverse CV events. Most commonly this is based on angiographic findings and a measure of left ventricular (LV) systolic function (usually with echocardiography). In general, patients without significant coronary artery disease (CAD) and/or a normal left ventricular ejection fraction (LVEF) face lower future CV risk.[11,12] Ambulatory continuous ECG monitoring to assess the ST-segment is less frequently performed, but can be used for prognostication.[13]

Prior to beginning phase 2 of cardiac rehabilitation, a thorough history and physical examination is recommended. It is important to identify comorbidities that may impact physical activity and educational barriers that may impact learning. A review of current medical therapy is also recommended to ensure that appropriate medications are prescribed and that vaccinations (influenza and pneumococcal) are up to date.[14,15] Finally, a patient treatment plan should be created that prioritizes the participant's goals and outlines intervention strategies that are coordinated with the patient's primary care provider and cardiologist.

For many patients, a 12-lead ECG may be the only testing needed prior to starting rehabilitation sessions. For ACS patients, however, stress testing may be recommended to provide an exercise prescription that defines the mode, frequency, duration, and intensity of exercise as well as the attendant risks.[16] This may be more important for patients with obstructive CAD that either have not undergone revascularization or were incompletely revascularized.

Nutritional Counseling

Nearly all patients have something to learn about how to improve their diet following an ACS. An inventory of caloric intake (i.e., types of foods habitually eaten) and content (i.e., saturated fat, *trans* fat, cholesterol, sodium, and nutrients), the number of meals and snacks, the location of meals (at home versus eating out), and the amount of alcohol consumed should all be part of the initial assessment for cardiac rehabilitation.[10] Attention should also be paid to comorbidities that may impact the type of nutritional intervention, such as diabetes mellitus (DM), hypertension, heart failure, or chronic kidney disease. Finally, family members should be included in education and counseling sessions to improve long-term compliance.

The recent 2013 AHA/American College of Cardiology (ACC) Lifestyle Management Guideline makes specific dietary recommendations to achieve blood pressure and low-density lipoprotein (LDL)-cholesterol goals (**Table 10.2**).[17]

Weight Management

Numerous studies have demonstrated a direct relationship between increasing body mass index (BMI) and waist circumference and the risks of CV disease,[18,19] type 2 DM,[19,20] and all-cause mortality.[21] For at-risk patients (BMI >25 kg/m^2 and/or a waist circumference >40 inches for men and >35 inches for women), reasonable short-term and long-term weight loss goals should be identified and implemented through a behavior program that combines dietary changes and physical activity. The recent 2013 AHA/ACC/The Obesity Society (TOS) Guideline for the Management of Overweight and Obesity in Adults makes specific dietary, counseling, and surgical recommendations to achieve these goals (**Table 10.3**).[22] Additional information on nutrition can also be found in the chapter on Lifestyle Modification.

Table 10.2
2013 AHA/ACC Lifestyle Management Guideline Dietary Recommendations[17]

Lifestyle recommendations for LDL-cholesterol lowering	COR/LOE
1. Consume a dietary pattern that emphasizes intake of vegetables, fruits, and whole grains; includes low-fat dairy products, poultry, fish, legumes, non-tropical vegetable oils and nuts; and limits intake of sweets, sugar-sweetened beverages, and red meats. • Adapt this dietary pattern to appropriate calorie requirements, personal and cultural food preferences, and nutrition therapy for other medical conditions (including diabetes mellitus). • Achieve this pattern by following plans such as the DASH dietary pattern, the USDA Food Pattern, or the AHA Diet.	Class I, Level A
2. Aim for a dietary pattern that achieves 5%–6% of calories from saturated fat.	Class I, Level A
3. Reduce percent of calories from saturated fat.	Class I, Level A
4. Reduce percent of calories from *trans* fat.	Class I, Level A
Lifestyle recommendations for blood pressure lowering	COR/LOE
1. Consume a dietary pattern that emphasizes intake of vegetables, fruits, and whole grains; includes low-fat dairy products, poultry, fish, legumes, non-tropical vegetable oils and nuts; and limits intake of sweets, sugar-sweetened beverages, and red meats. • Adapt this dietary pattern to appropriate calorie requirements, personal and cultural food preferences, and nutrition therapy for other medical conditions (including diabetes mellitus). • Achieve this pattern by following plans such as the DASH dietary pattern, the USDA Food Pattern, or the AHA Diet.	Class I, Level A
2. Lower sodium intake.	Class I, Level A
3. Consume no more than 2400 mg of sodium per day.	Class IIa, Level B

AHA = American Heart Association, DASH = dietary approaches to stop hypertension, COR = class of recommendation, LDL = low-density lipoprotein, LOE = level of evidence, USDA = U.S. Department of Agriculture.

Table 10.3
2013 AHA/ACC/TOS Guideline for the Management of Overweight and Obesity in Adults Recommendations[22]

Diets for weight loss	COR/LOE
1. Prescribe a diet to achieve reduced calorie intake for obese or overweight individuals who would benefit from weight loss, as part of a comprehensive lifestyle intervention with 1 of the following: • 1200–1500 kcal/day for women and 1500–1800 kcal/day for men. • 500–750 kcal/day energy deficit. • Use one of the evidence-based diets that restricts certain food types (e.g., high-carbohydrate foods, low-fiber foods, or high-fat foods) in order to create an energy deficit by reduced food intake.	Class I, Level A
2. Prescribe a calorie-restricted diet for obese or overweight individuals who would benefit from weight loss, based on the patient's preferences and health status, and preferably refer to a nutrition professional for counseling.	Class I, Level A
Lifestyle interventions and counseling for weight loss	**COR/LOE**
1. Advise participation in a comprehensive lifestyle program that assists participants in adhering to a lower calorie diet and increasing physical activity through the use of behavioral strategies.	Class I, Level A
2. Prescribe on-site, high-intensity (i.e., ≥14 sessions in 6 months) comprehensive weight loss interventions provided in individual or group sessions by a trained interventionist.	Class I, Level A
3. Consider prescription of electronically delivered weight loss programs (including by telephone) that includes personalized feedback from a trained interventionist, recognizing that it may result in smaller weight loss than face-to-face interventions.	Class IIa, Level A
4. Consider some commercial-based programs that provide comprehensive lifestyle interventions, provided there is peer-reviewed published evidence of their safety and efficacy.	Class IIa, Level A

(Continued)

Table 10.3 (Continued)	
5. Consider a very low calorie diet (<800 kcal/day) only in limited circumstances and only when provided by trained practitioners in a medical care setting where medical monitoring and high-intensity lifestyle intervention can be provided.	Class IIa, Level A
6. Advise individuals who have lost weight to participate long term (≥1 year) in a comprehensive weight loss maintenance program.	Class I, Level A
7. Prescribe face-to-face or telephone-delivered weight loss maintenance programs that provide regular contact (≥ monthly) with a trained interventionist who helps participants engage in high levels of physical activity (i.e., 200–300 minutes/week), monitor body weight regularly (≥ weekly), and consume a reduced-calorie diet (need to lower body weight).	Class I, Level A
Selection criteria for bariatric surgical treatment of obesity	COR/LOE
1. Advise adults with a BMI ≥40 kg/m^2 or BMI ≥35 kg/m^2 with obesity-related comorbid conditions who are motivated to lose weight and who have not responded to behavioral treatment with or without pharmacotherapy with sufficient weight loss to achieve targeted health outcome goals that bariatric surgery may be an appropriate option to improve health and offer referral to an experienced bariatric surgeon for consultation and evaluation.	Class IIa, Level A

BMI = body mass index, COR = class of recommendation, LOE = level of evidence.

Blood Pressure Management

Hypertension is one of the most prevalent CV risk factors worldwide. It is associated with a number of adverse CV events, including an increased risk of a first and subsequent myocardial infarction (MI).[23,24] Blood pressure lowering agents are routinely administered to patients following an ACS, usually in the form of BBs and inhibitors of the renin-angiotensin system (i.e., ACE inhibitors or angiotensin receptor blockers).

A blood pressure goal of <130/80 mmHg was traditionally recommended for patients with CAD, however, several trials called this cut point into question.[25,26] This lent support in 2014 to change the goal to <140/90 mmHg, with a liberalized goal of <150/90 mmHg at an older age (≥60 years in the U.S. guidelines and >80 years in the European guidelines).[27–29] This is now questioned by the recently halted SPRINT trial, which demonstrated significantly reduced rates of death and CV events among those ≥50 years with additional CV risk factors (not diabetes) receiving more intensive blood pressure control (systolic blood pressure <120 mmHg vs. 140 mmHg).[30] These recent findings will almost certainly impact upcoming recommendations when the new ACC/AHA Hypertension Guidelines are released in 2016.

Beyond pharmacotherapy, several lifestyle interventions have been associated with notable reductions in systolic blood pressure (**Table 10.2** and **Table 10.4**). Nonprescription drugs that may adversely affect blood pressure should also be avoided (i.e., nonsteroidal anti-inflammatory drugs).[31] Initial assessment of blood pressure in both arms at program entry and regular assessment in at least one arm during subsequent visits is important to assess ongoing treatment compliance.[10] Adjustment of antihypertensive therapy should be performed in coordination with the patient's primary care provider and/or cardiologist.

Lipid Management

A fasting lipid panel is recommended for all ACS patients. Abnormal levels of lipoproteins (LDL-cholesterol, high-density lipoprotein [HDL]-cholesterol, and triglyceride) are strongly associated with the development and progression of CV disease.[32–34] LDL-cholesterol serves as the primary focus of current guideline recommendations given the preponderance of randomized controlled trial data supporting its reduction

Table 10.4
2013 AHA/ACC/Centers for Disease Control (CDC) Lifestyle Modifications for Treatment of Hypertension[28]

Lifestyle Modification	Recommendation	Approximate SBP Reduction (Range)
Reduce weight	• Maintain normal body weight (body mass index of 18.5–24.9 kg/m^2).	5–20 mmHg/10 kg weight loss
Adopt DASH eating plan	• Consume a diet rich in fruits, vegetables, and low-fat dairy products with a reduced content of saturated and total fat.	8–14 mmHg
Lower sodium intake	• Consume no more than 2400 mg of sodium/day. • Further reduce sodium intake to 1500 mg/day. • Reduce intake of sodium by at least 1000 mg/day even if the desired daily sodium intake is not achieved.	2–8 mmHg
Physical activity	Engage in regular aerobic physical activity such as brisk walking (at least 30 minutes per day most days of the week).	4–9 mmHg
Moderation of alcohol consumption	Limit consumption to no more than 2 drinks (e.g., 24 oz beer, 10 oz wine, or 3 oz of 80-proof alcohol) per day in most men and no more than 1 drink per day in women and light-weight individuals.	2–4 mmHg

DASH = dietary approaches to stop hypertension, SBP = systolic blood pressure.

in at-risk populations.[35] Beyond lifestyle recommendations (Table 10.2), statins are unequivocally the preferred drug to lower LDL-cholesterol levels.[36]

Based on the recent cholesterol guidelines,[35] a high-intensity statin is recommended for patients with established atherosclerotic CV disease (ASCVD).[35] A moderate-intensity statin (Table 10.5) should be considered for individuals

Table 10.5
High- and Moderate-Intensity Statin Regimens[35]

High-intensity Statin Therapy (daily dose lowers LDL-cholesterol by approximately ≥50%)	Moderate-intensity Statin Therapy (daily dose lowers LDL-cholesterol by approximately 30% to <50%)
Atorvastatin 40–80 mg	Atorvastatin 10–20 mg
Rosuvastatin 20–40 mg	Fluvastatin XL 80 mg
	Fluvastatin 40 mg twice daily
	Lovastatin 40 mg
	Pitavastatin 2–4 mg
	Pravastatin 40–80 mg
	Rosuvastatin 5–10 mg
	Simvastatin 20–40 mg

>75 years or in those unable to take a high-intensity statin.[35] For patients tolerant of the initial recommended statin regimen, continued adherence should be regularly reinforced with a follow-up fasting lipid panel in 1–3 months. Additional lipid testing should be performed every 3–12 months thereafter. Earlier follow up (1–3 months) is recommended for patients intolerant of the recommended statin regimen, with dose or medication adjustment as necessary.

Diabetes Management

Not only is DM a potent risk factor for the development of CV disease, it also significantly increases the risk of recurrent CV events.[37–40] While diabetic patients with MI tend to be older with greater numbers of comorbidities, increased risk persists even after adjusting for these factors. Current guidelines recommend a hemoglobin $A1_C$ <7.0% for most,[41,42] reserving a target of <7.5%–8.0% for frail older adults and/or those with a life expectancy of <5 years.[41,43]

As part of the initial evaluation, the signs and symptoms of both hypoglycemia and hyperglycemia should be assessed. For those taking insulin or insulin secretagogues, it is important to 1) avoid exercising at times of peak insulin, 2) check blood sugar levels both pre- and post-exercise, 3) encourage adequate hydration to avoid fluid shifts that can affect blood sugar levels, and 4) educate patients that blood sugar levels may continue to fall for 24–48 hours after exercise.[10] Prior to exercise, if blood sugar levels are <100 mg/dL, exercise should be postponed, 15 grams of carbohydrate should be consumed, and blood sugar levels should be retested in 15 minutes.[10] In contrast, if pre-exercise blood sugar levels are >300 mg/dL, exercise can be pursued as long as the patient feels well, is adequately hydrated, and there is no evidence of blood or urinary ketones.[10]

For patients taking other oral hypoglycemic agents, it is recommended that pre-exercise blood sugar levels be checked for the first 6–10 rehabilitation sessions, primarily to assess the degree of glycemic control.[10] Exercise-induced hypoglycemia is unlikely with these agents. All cases of hypoglycemia or hyperglycemia should be reported to the patient's primary care provider and/or endocrinologist in order to modify the patient's treatment regimen.

Tobacco Cessation

Tobacco is a potent contributor to initial and recurrent CV events,[23,44] with cigarettes accounting for greater than one-third of CV deaths in the United States.[45] Though not as well studied, there appears to be similar increased risk with cigar,[46] pipe,[47] and smokeless tobacco[48] as well.

Because tobacco cessation is associated with substantial CV benefit,[49-51] it is important to regularly assess readiness at rehabilitation encounters. It is recommended to use the 5 R's[52] when patients are not ready to quit and the 5 As when they are[53] (**Table 10.6**). Patients should always be encouraged to avoid exposure to second-hand smoke at work and at home.

Both behavioral counseling and pharmacotherapy increase the rate of smoking cessation and are additive if combined.[54,55] Alternative options with varied success include acupuncture, aversive therapy, financial incentives, and hypnotherapy. Even though 1-year abstinence rates approximate only 30% with optimal therapy,[56] smokers should still be strongly motivated to quit, as continued tobacco abuse is associated with a lower likelihood of completing cardiac rehabilitation.

Table 10.6
5 Rs and 5 As of Smoking Cessation[52,53]

5 Rs for Patients Not Ready to Quit
1. Relevance—Encourage the patient to indicate why quitting is personally relevant.
2. Risks—Ask the patient to identify potential negative consequences of tobacco use.
3. Rewards—Ask the patient to identify potential benefits of stopping tobacco use.
4. Roadblocks—Ask the patient to identify barriers or impediments to quitting.
5. Repetition—The motivational intervention should be repeated every time an unmotivated patient has an interaction with a clinician. Tobacco users who have failed in previous quit attempts should be told that most people make repeated quit attempts before they are successful.

5 As for Patients Who Are Ready to Quit
1. Ask—Systematically identify all tobacco users at every visit.
2. Advise—Strongly urge all smokers to quit.
3. Assess—Identify smokers willing to make a quit attempt.
4. Assist—Aid the patient in quitting.
5. Arrange—Schedule follow-up contact.

Psychosocial Management

An ACS represents a major life-changing event for most patients. On top of this, several personality and mood disorders have been identified as contributors to increased CV risk.[57] Acute and chronic stress, hostility, cynicism, and anger likely do this (at least in part) through activation of the sympathetic nervous system. Anxiety and depression also contribute; however, the underlying mechanisms are less well understood.

Over 15% of patients experience major depression early after an MI and >30% will have significant depressive symptoms.[58] Other psychosocial stressors (i.e., hostility, social isolation, anxiety, anger, and marital stress) are associated with a poor prognosis after an MI, likely from poor compliance with risk-reducing interventions. In spite of this, there are some data suggesting benefit from psychotherapy and/or pharmacotherapy in treating depressive symptoms.[59–61]

Individualized and/or small group education should be held on stress management, mindfulness, and adjusting to a life with heart disease. Family members should be included in the discussion when possible to facilitate a strong social support system. Some patients will require specialized behavioral health therapy that should be coordinated by the patient's primary care provider.

Physical Activity Counseling and Exercise Training

Exercise represents physical activity that is regular, purposeful, and aimed at promoting fitness. It has a favorable effect on multiple health outcomes and is strongly recommended for patients with established CV disease.[62] Beyond weight control, exercise improves lipid parameters,[63] blood pressure,[64] glycemic control,[65] and psychological health.[66]

Assessment of occupational, recreational, and daily living physical activity needs is an important first step in

Table 10.7
Aerobic and Resistance Exercise Recommendations[10]

	Aerobic exercise	Resistance exercise
Frequency	3–5 days/week	2–3 days/week
Intensity	50%–80% of exercise capacity	10–15 repetitions/set to moderate fatigue
Duration	20–60 minutes	1–3 sets of 8–10 upper and lower body exercises
Modalities	Examples include walking, treadmill, cycling, rowing, stair climbing, and arm/leg ergometry	Examples include calisthenics, elastic bands, cuff/hand weights, dumbbells, free weights, wall pulleys, and weight machines

rehabilitation. Barriers to physical activity should be identified, and social support systems as well as assist devices should be leveraged. For most ACS patients, a symptom-limited stress test can help provide an exercise prescription that safely defines the frequency, intensity, and duration of exercise that should be sought.[16]

For most patients, a combination of aerobic and resistance (strength) exercise is recommended (**Table 10.7**).[10] Warm-up activities, cool-downs, and flexibility exercises should be incorporated into all sessions. Exercise progression should be modified based on regular reassessment.

THE CLINICAL BENEFITS ASSOCIATED WITH CARDIAC REHABILITATION

Benefits associated with cardiac rehabilitation are numerous and manifest both in the short- and long-term. Beyond hemodynamic improvement (lower double product with peak exercise and improved heart rate recovery), participation in cardiac rehabilitation is associated with significantly lower rates of recurrent adverse CV events.[67,68]

In 2004, a meta-analysis of 48 trials with 8940 patients sought to evaluate the effect of cardiac rehabilitation following coronary revascularization (mostly in patients with a recent ACS). Compared with usual care, treatment with cardiac rehabilitation was associated with a significant reduction in cardiac (OR = 0.74, 95% CI 0.61–0.96) and all-cause (OR = 0.80, 95% CI = 0.68–0.93) mortality.[69] A 2011 follow up meta-analysis of 34 trials with 6111 post-MI patients confirmed these findings in a more contemporary cohort. Patients randomized to exercise-based cardiac rehabilitation experienced a lower risk of reinfarction (OR = 0.53, 95% CI 0.38–0.76), cardiac mortality (OR = 0.64, 95% CI 0.46–0.88), and all-cause mortality (OR = 0.74, 95% CI 0.58–0.95).[70]

Benefits associated with cardiac rehabilitation are directly related to the number of sessions completed. In an observational analysis of 30,161 Medicare beneficiaries that participated in at least 1 session of cardiac rehabilitation, attendance at 36 sessions (perfect attendance) was associated with a lower risk of MI and death compared to that of patients attending 24 sessions (OR = 0.88, 95% CI 0.83–0.93 for MI; OR = 0.86, 95% CI 0.77–0.97 for death), 12 sessions (OR = 0.77, 95% CI 0.69–0.87 for MI; OR = 0.78, 95% CI 0.71–0.87 for death), and 1 session (OR = 0.69, 95% CI 0.58–0.81 for MI; OR = 0.53, 95% CI 0.48–0.59 for death).[71] A follow-up prospective study of 5886 Canadian patients referred for cardiac rehabilitation (70% following an ACS) compared 2900 patients that completed the program to 554 that started but did not finish the program and 2432 that never started at all. Compared with nonstarters and partial completers, those who finished the entire program had a lower risk of all-cause hospitalization (OR = 0.77, 95% CI 0.71–0.84) and death (OR = 0.59, 95% CI 0.49–0.84).[72]

Many benefits associated with cardiac rehabilitation diminish if healthful behaviors are not maintained over time.

In a prospective cohort study of 2441 patients who completed cardiac rehabilitation, rates of tobacco use, hypertension, and dyslipidemia fell significantly after completion of the program (tobacco use fell from 39% to 5%; hypertension fell from 24% to 8%; and dyslipidemia fell from 57% to 29%), but increased significantly at 12 months (tobacco use rose from 5% to 10%; hypertension rose from 8% to 25%; and dyslipidemia rose from 29% to 51%).[73] As such, it is critical that providers reinforce diet, exercise, stress relief, and healthful behaviors at every visit.

THE MYTHS UNDERLYING CARDIAC REHABILITATION'S UNDERUTILIZATION

Cardiac rehabilitation represents one of the most effective risk-reducing interventions following an ACS. According to the Agency for Healthcare Research and Quality (AHRQ), it improves processes of care, enhances quality of life and functional status, and leads to reductions in the rates of hospitalization, recurrent MI, and long-term mortality.[7] In spite of this, it is vastly underutilized, with fewer than 20% of eligible individuals participating in cardiac rehabilitation after a MI.[5,6] Several misconceptions likely underlie this.

Cardiac Rehabilitation Is Not Safe

By far, the benefits associated with supervised exercise exceed any attendant risks. In a study of 25,420 patients who underwent 743,471 patient-hours of exercise training, adverse cardiac events were reported at a rate of 1 per 49,565 hours exercised.[74] In addition, cardiac arrest occurred at a rate of 1.3 per million hours exercised, and no fatal events were reported.

Cardiac Rehabilitation Is Not Appropriate for Older Adults

More than 50% of patients with an ACS are ≥65 years of age. Many of the benefits associated with cardiac rehabilitation are similar between individuals of younger and older ages[75–77]; however, older individuals (along with women, non-Caucasians, and the uninsured) are less likely to be referred.[78] ACS-related complications (including deconditioning) occur more commonly in those at an older age, and thus underscore the importance of cardiac rehabilitation in this group.[79] Greater attention should be spent on warm-ups and cool-downs as well as flexibility to minimize injury and/or adverse hemodynamic effects.

Cardiac Rehabilitation Is Not Covered by Insurance

Current guidelines recommend cardiac rehabilitation as first-line therapy for patients with varied forms of CAD, including those with an ACS, chronic stable angina, and/or those who have undergone percutaneous or surgical revascularization. In 2006, Medicare deemed cardiac rehabilitation reasonable and necessary for these conditions.[80] Based on this, most payers have followed suit.

Cardiac Rehabilitation Is Not Cost-Effective

Numerous studies have suggested that cardiac rehabilitation is a cost-effective intervention following an ACS. Reported incremental cost-effectiveness ratios have ranged from $4400 to $13,600 per quality-adjusted life-year saved.[81–83]

These benefits also extend over the long term. In a retrospective analysis of 2395 patients who underwent percutaneous coronary intervention (mostly for a recent ACS), participation in cardiac rehabilitation was associated with a significant reduction in all-cause mortality (HR = 0.54, 95% CI 0.41–0.71, $p < 0.001$). The numbers needed to treat to prevent 1 death were 34 and 22 at 1 and 5 years, respectively.[84] In a similar analysis of 846 patients who underwent coronary artery bypass graft surgery (CABG), participation in cardiac rehabilitation was associated with a significant reduction in all-cause mortality (HR = 0.54, 95% CI 0.40–0.74, $p < 0.001$), with a number needed to treat of only 8 over 10 years.[85]

Cardiac Rehabilitation Programs Are Not Conveniently Located

Obviously cardiac rehabilitation programs are only likely to be used if they are accessible. The AACVPR has 1691 programs listed in its searchable database[86]; however, this is likely an underestimation of the total number of available programs. Unfortunately, these programs are not uniformly distributed relative to population or geography,[87] which can contribute to underutilization.

Patients are less likely to enroll in cardiac rehabilitation programs when they have to drive more than 30–60 minutes to the closest program.[88,89] For these individuals, however, telehealth-, community-, or home-based cardiac rehabilitation programs should be considered.[90]

CONCLUSION

Cardiac rehabilitation is a highly effective intervention with very favorable near- and long-term CV effects following an ACS. Unfortunately, it is disappointingly underutilized. Program access is often blamed as a major barrier to participation; however, it is much more commonly due to limited knowledge and/or skepticism by providers.[91] An improved understanding of what cardiac rehabilitation offers, the automation of referral at the time of hospital discharge, and inclusion of nonphysician providers in the referral process can all significantly improve participation. If we are sincerely dedicated to reducing future CV risk, this is the least that we can do for our patients.

REFERENCES

1. Go AS, Mozaffarian D, Roger VL, et al., Heart Disease and Stroke Statistics—2013 Update: A report from the American Heart Association. *Circulation.* 2013;127:e6–e245.
2. Gluckman TJ, Sachdev M, Schulman SP, Blumenthal RS. A simplified approach to the management of non-ST-segment elevation acute coronary syndromes. *JAMA.* 2005;293:349–357.
3. Hamm CW, Bassand JP, Agewall S, et al. ESC Guidelines for the management of acute coronary syndromes in patients presenting without persistent ST-segment elevation: The Task Force for the management of acute coronary syndromes (ACS) in patients presenting without persistent ST-segment elevation of the European Society of Cardiology (ASC). *Eur Heart J.* 2011;32:2999–3054.
4. Ford ES, Ajani UA, Croft JB, et al. Explaining the decrease in U.S. deaths from coronary disease, 1980–2000. *N Engl J Med.* 2007;356:2388–2398.
5. Cottin Y, Cambou JP, Casillas JM, Ferrières J, Cantet C, Danchin N. Specific profile and referral bias of rehabilitated patients after an acute coronary syndrome. *J Cardiopulm Rehabil.* 2004;24:38–44.
6. Suaya JA, Shepard DS, Normand SL, Ades PA, Prottas J, Stason WB. Use of cardiac rehabilitation by Medicare beneficiaries after myocardial infarction or coronary bypass surgery. *Circulation.* 2007;116:1653–1662.
7. Wenger NK, Froelicher ES, Smith LK, et al. *Cardiac Rehabilitation: Clinical Practice Guideline No. 17.* Rockville, MD: U.S. Dept of Health and Human Services, Public Health Service, Agency for Health Care Policy and Research, National Heart, Lung, and Blood Institute; October 1995. AHCPR publication No. 96-0672.
8. O'Gara PT, Kushner FG, Ascheim DD, et al. 2013 ACCF/AHA guideline for the management of ST-elevation myocardial infarction: A report of the American College of Cardiology Foundation/American Heart Association Task Force on Practice Guidelines. *J Am Coll Cardiol.* 2013;61:e78–e140.
9. Anderson JL, Adams CD, Antman EM, et al. 2012 ACCF/AHA focused update incorporated into the ACCF/AHA 2007 guidelines

for the management of patients with unstable angina/non-ST-elevation myocardial infarction: A report of the American College of Cardiology Foundation/American Heart Association Task Force on Practice Guideline. *J Am Coll Cardiol.* 2013;61:e179–e347.

10. Balady GJ, Williams MA, Ades PA, et al. Core components of cardiac rehabilitation/secondary prevention programs: 2007 update: A Scientific Statement from the American Heart Association Exercise, Cardiac Rehabilitation, and Prevention Committee, the Council on Clinical Cardiology; the Councils on Cardiovascular Nursing, Epidemiology and Prevention, and Nutrition, Physical Activity, and Metabolism; and the American Association of Cardiovascular and Pulmonary Rehabilitation. *Circulation.* 2007;115:2675–2682.
11. Bugiardini R, Manfrini O, De Ferrari GM. Unanswered questions for management of acute coronary syndrome: Risk stratification of patients with minimal disease or normal findings on coronary angiography. *Arch Intern Med.* 2006;166:1391–1395.
12. Burns RJ, Gibbons RJ, Yi Q, et al. The relationships of left ventricular ejection fraction, end-systolic volume index and infarct size to six-month mortality after hospital discharge following myocardial infarction treated by thrombolysis. *J Am Coll Cardiol.* 2002;39:30–36.
13. Scirica BM, Morrow DA, Budaj A, et al. Ischemia detected on continuous electrocardiography after acute coronary syndrome: Observations from the MERLIN-TIMI 36 (Metabolic Efficiency With Ranolazine for Less Ischemia in Non-ST-Elevation Acute Coronary Syndrome-Thrombolysis in Myocardial Infarction 36) trial. *J Am Coll Cardiol.* 2009;53:1411–1421.
14. Nichol KL, Nordin J, Mullooly J, Lask R, Fillbrandt K, Iwane M. Influenza vaccination and reduction in hospitalizations for cardiac disease and stroke among the elderly. *N Engl J Med.* 2003;348:1322–1332.
15. Udell JA, Zawi R, Bhatt DL, et al. Association between influenza vaccination and cardiovascular outcomes in high-risk patients: A meta-analysis. *JAMA.* 2013;310:1711–1720.
16. Thompson PD. Exercise prescription and proscription for patients with coronary artery disease. *Circulation.* 2005;112:2354–2363.
17. Eckel RH, Jakicic JM, Ard JD, et al. 2013 AHA/ACC guideline on lifestyle management to reduce cardiovascular risk: A report of the American College of Cardiology/American Heart Association Task Force on Practice Guidelines. *J Am Coll Cardiol.* 2014;63(25 Pt B):2960–2984.
18. Ni Mhurchu C, Rodgers A, Pan WH, et al. Body mass index and cardiovascular disease in the Asia-Pacific region: An overview of 33 cohorts involving 310,000 participants. *Int J Epidemiol.* 2004;33:751–758.
19. Janssen I, Katzmarzyk PT, Ross R. Body mass index, waist circumference, and health risk: Evidence in support of current National Institutes of Health guidelines. *Arch Intern Med.* 2002;162:2074–2079.

20. Bays HE, Chapman RH, Grandy S. The relationship of body mass index to diabetes mellitus, hypertension and dyslipideaemia: Comparison of data from two national surveys. *Int J Clin Pract.* 2007;61:737–747.

21. Whitlock G, Lewington S, Sherliker P, et al. Body-mass index and cause-specific mortality in 900,000 adults: Collaborative analyses of 57 prospective studies. *Lancet.* 2009;373:1083–1096.

22. Jensen MD, Ryan DH, Apovian CM, et al. 2013 AHA/ACC/TOS guideline for the management of overweight and obesity in adults: A report of the American College of Cardiology/American Heart Association Task Force on Practice Guidelines and the Obesity Society. *J Am Coll Cardiol.* 2014;63(25 Pt B):2985–3023.

23. Yusuf S, Hawken S, Ounpuu S, et al. Effect of potentially modifiable risk factors associated with myocardial infarction in 52 countries (the INTERHEART study): Case-control study. *Lancet.* 2004;364:937–952.

24. Lewington S, Clarke R, Qizilbash, et al. Age-specific relevance of usual blood pressure to vascular mortality: A meta-analysis of individual data for one million adults in 61 prospective studies. *Lancet.* 2002;360:1903–1913.

25. Zanchetti A, Grassi G, Mancia G. When should antihypertensive drug treatment be initiated and to what levels should systolic blood pressure be lowered? A critical reappraisal. *J Hypertens.* 2009;27:923–934.

26. Czernichow S, Zanchetti A, Turnbull F, et al. The effects of blood pressure reduction and of different blood pressure-lowering regimens on major cardiovascular events according to baseline blood pressure: meta-analysis of randomized trials. *J Hypertens.* 2011;29:4–16.

27. Mancia G, Fargard R, Narkiewicz K, et al. 2013 ESH/ESC guidelines for the management of arterial hypertension: The Task Force for the Management of Arterial Hypertension of the European Society of Hypertension (ESH) and of the European Society of Cardiology (ESC). *Eur Heart J.* 2013;34:2159–2219.

28. Go AS, Bauman MA, Coleman King SM, et al. An effective approach to high blood pressure control: A science advisory from the American Heart Association, the American College of Cardiology, and the Centers for Disease Control and Prevention. *J Am Coll Cardiol.* 2014;63:1230–1238.

29. James PA, Oparil S, Carter BL, et al. 2014 evidence-based guideline for the management of high blood pressure in adults: Report from the panel members appointed to the Eighth Joint National Committee (JNC 8). *JAMA.* 2014;311:507–520.

30. Wright JT, Jr., Williamson JD, Whelton PK, et al. A randomized trial of intensive versus standard blood-pressure control. *N Engl J Med.* 2015;373:2103–2116.

31. Chobanian AV, Bakris GL, Black HR, et al. The Seventh Report of the Joint National Committee on Prevention, Detection, Evaluation, and Treatment of High Blood Pressure: The JNC 7 report. *JAMA*. 2003;289:2560–2572.
32. Grundy SM, Cleeman JI, Merz CN, et al. Implications of recent clinical trials for the National Cholesterol Education Program Adult Treatment Panel III Guidelines. *Circulation*. 2004;110:227–239.
33. Kannel WB. High-density lipoproteins: Epidemiologic profile and risks of coronary artery disease. *Am J Cardiol*. 1983;52:9B–12B.
34. Sarwar N, Danesh J, Eiriksdottir G, et al. Triglycerides and the risk of coronary heart disease: 10,158 incident cases among 262,525 participants in 29 Western prospective studies. *Circulation*. 2007;115:450–458.
35. Stone NJ, Robinson JG, Lichtenstein AH, et al. 2013 ACC/AHA guideline on the treatment of blood cholesterol to reduce atherosclerotic cardiovascular risk in adults: A report of the American College of Cardiology/American Heart Association Task Force on Practice Guidelines. *J Am Coll Cardiol*. 2014;63(25 Pt B):2889–2934.
36. Baigent C, Blackwell L, Emberson J, et al. Efficacy and safety of more intensive lowering of LDL cholesterol: A meta-analysis of data from 170,000 participants in 26 randomised trials. *Lancet*. 2010;376:1670–1681.
37. Haffner SM, Lehto S, Rönnemaa T, Pyörälä K, Laakso M. Mortality from coronary heart disease in subjects with type 2 diabetes and in nondiabetic subjects with and without prior myocardial infarction. *N Engl J Med*. 1998;339:229–234.
38. Lee CD, Folsom AR, Pankow JS, Brancati FL. Cardiovascular events in diabetic and nondiabetic adults with or without history of myocardial infarction. *Circulation*. 2004;109:855–860.
39. Malik S, Wong ND, Franklin SS, et al. Impact of the metabolic syndrome on mortality from coronary heart disease, cardiovascular disease, and all causes in United States adults. *Circulation*. 2004;110:1245–1250.
40. Sarwar N, Gao P, Seshasai SR, et al. Diabetes mellitus, fasting blood glucose concentration, and risk of vascular disease: A collaborative meta-analysis of 102 prospective studies. *Lancet*. 2010;375:2215–2222.
41. Inzucchi SE, Bergenstal RM, Buse JB, et al. Management of hyperglycemia in type 2 diabetes: A patient-centered approach: Position statement of the American Diabetes Association (ADA) and the European Association for the Study of Diabetes (EASD). *Diabetes Care*. 2012;35:1364–1379.
42. Rydén L, Grant PJ, Anker SD, et al. ESC Guidelines on diabetes, pre-diabetes, and cardiovascular diseases developed in collaboration with the EASD: The Task Force on diabetes, pre-diabetes,

and cardiovascular diseases of the European Society of Cardiology (ESC) and developed in collaboration with the European Association for the Study of Diabetes (EASD). *Eur Heart J.* 20143;34: 3035–3087.

43. Huang ES, Zhang Q, Gandra N, Chin MH, Meltzer DO. The effect of comorbid illness and functional status on the expected benefits of intensive glucose control in older patients with type 2 diabetes: A decision analysis. *Ann Intern Med.* 2008;149:11–19.
44. Tofler GH, Muller JE, Stone PH, Davies G, Davis VG, Braunwald E. Comparison of long-term outcome after myocardial infarction in patients never graduated from high school with that in more educated patients. Multicenter Investigation of the Limitation of Infarct Size (MILIS). *Am J Cardiol.* 1993;71:1031–1035.
45. Chapter 6: Cardiovascular diseases. In: *A Report of the Surgeon General: How Tobacco Smoke Causes Disease: The Biology and Behavioral Basis for Smoking-Attributable Disease: A Report of the Surgeon General.* Centers for Disease Control and Prevention; National Center for Chronic Disease Prevention and Health Promotion; Office on Smoking and Health. Atlanta, GA: Centers for Disease Control and Prevention; 2010. Available at: http://www.ncbi.nlm.nih.gov/books/NBK53012/. Accessed December 11, 2015.
46. Jacobs EJ, Thun MJ, Apicella LF. Cigar smoking and death from coronary heart disease in a prospective study of U.S. men. *Arch Intern Med.* 1999;159:2413–2418.
47. Tverdal A, Bjartveit K. Health consequences of pipe versus cigarette smoking. *Tob Control.* 2011;20:123–130.
48. Bolinder G, Alfredsson L, Englund A, de Faire U. Smokeless tobacco use and increased cardiovascular mortality among Swedish construction workers. *Am J Public Health.* 1994;84:399–404.
49. Wilson K, Gibson N, Willan A, Cook D. Effect of smoking cessation on mortality after myocardial infarction: Meta-analysis of cohort studies. *Arch Intern Med.* 2000;160:939–944.
50. Critchley JA, Capewell S. Mortality risk reduction associated with smoking cessation in patients with coronary heart disease: A systematic review. *JAMA.* 2003;290:86–97.
51. Critchley J, Capewell S. Smoking cessation for the secondary prevention of coronary heart disease. *Cochrane Database Syst Rev.* 2004;(1):CD003041. Review.
52. *Patients Not Ready To Make A Quit Attempt Now (The "5 R's").* Dec 2012. Rockville, MD: Agency for Healthcare Research and Quality. Available at http://www.ahrq.gov/professionals/clinicians-providers/guidelines-recommendations/tobacco/5rs.html. Accessed December 11, 2015.
53. Fiore MC, Bailey WC, Cohen SJ, et al. *Smoking Cessation. Clinical Practice Guideline No. 18.* Rockville, MD: U.S. Department of Health

and Human Services, Public Health Service, Agency for Health Care Policy and Research. AHCPR Publication No. 96-0692. Apr 1996.

54. Fiore MC, Jaén CR, Baker TB, et al. Clinical Practice Guideline: Treating tobacco use and dependence: 2008 update. Rockville, MD: U.S. Department of Health and Human Services, 2008. Available at http://bphc.hrsa.gov/buckets/treatingtobacco.pdf. Accessed December 11, 2015.
55. Silagy C, Lancaster T, Stead L, Mant D, Fowler G. Nicotine replacement therapy for smoking cessation. *Cochrane Database Syst Rev.* 2002;(4):CD000146.
56. Rigotti NA. Clinical practice. Treatment of tobacco use and dependence. *N Engl J Med.* 2002;346:506–512.
57. Rosengren A, Hawken S, Ounpuu S, et al. Association of psychosocial risk factors with risk of acute myocardial infarction in 11,119 cases and 13,648 controls from 52 countries (the INTERHEART study): Case-control study. *Lancet.* 2004;364:953–962.
58. Ziegelstein RC. Depression in patients recovering from a myocardial infarction. *JAMA.* 2001;286;1621–1627.
59. Glassman AH, O'Connor CM, Califf RM, et al. Sertraline treatment of major depression in patients with acute MI or unstable angina. *JAMA.* 2002;288:701–709.
60. Berkman LF, Blumentyhal J, Burg M, et al. Effects of treating depression and low perceived social support on clinical events after myocardial infarction: The Enhancing Recovery in Coronary Heart Disease Patients (ENRICHD) randomized trial. *JAMA.* 2003;289:3106–3116.
61. Lesperance F, Frasure-Smith N, Koszycki D, et al. Effects of citalopram and interpersonal psychotherapy on depression in patients with coronary artery disease: The Canadian Cardiac Randomized Evaluation of Antidepressant and Psychotherapy Efficacy (CREATE) trial. *JAMA.* 2007;297:367–397.
62. Wannamethee SG, Shaper AG, Walker M. Physical activity and mortality in older men with diagnosed coronary heart disease. *Circulation.* 2000;102:1358–1363.
63. Kraus WE, Houmard JA, Duscha BD, et al. Effects of the amount and intensity of exercise on plasma lipoproteins. *N Engl J Med.* 2002;347:1483–1492.
64. Whelton SP, Chin A, Xin X, He J. Effect of aerobic exercise on blood pressure: A meta-analysis of randomized, controlled trials. *Ann Intern Med.* 2002;136:493–503.
65. Umpierre D, Ribeiro PA, Kramer CK, et al. Physical activity advice only or structured exercise training and association with HbA1c levels in type 2 diabetes: A systematic review and meta-analysis. *JAMA.* 2011;305:1790–1799.
66. Martin CK, Church TS, Thompson AM, Earnest CP, Blair SN. Exercise dose and quality of life: A randomized controlled trial. *Arch Intern Med.* 2009;169:269–278.

67. Oldridge NB, Guyatt GH, Fischer ME, Rimm AA. Cardiac rehabilitation after myocardial infarction. Combined experience of randomized clinical trials. *JAMA*. 1988;260:945–950.
68. Clark AM, Hartling L, Vandermeer B, McAlister FA. Meta-analysis: Secondary prevention programs for patients with coronary artery disease. *Ann Intern Med*. 2005;143:659–672.
69. Taylor RS, Brown A, Ebrahim S, et al. Exercise-based rehabilitation for patients with coronary heart disease: Systematic review and meta-analysis of randomized controlled trials. *Am J Med*. 2004;116:682–692.
70. Lawler PR, Filion KB, Eisenberg MJ. Efficacy of exercise-based cardiac rehabilitation post-myocardial infarction: A systematic review and meta-analysis of randomized controlled trials. *Am Heart J*. 2011;162:571–584.
71. Hammill BG, Curtis LH, Schulman KA, Whellan DJ. Relationship between cardiac rehabilitation and long-term risks of death and myocardial infarction among elderly Medicare beneficiaries. *Circulation*. 2010;121:63–70.
72. Martin BJ, Hauer T, Arena R, et al. Cardiac rehabilitation attendance and outcomes in coronary artery disease patients. *Circulation*. 2012;126:677–687.
73. Willich SN, Müller-Nordhorn J, Kulig M, et al. Cardiac risk factors, medication, and recurrent clinical events after acute coronary disease; a prospective cohort study. *Eur Heart J*. 2001;22:307–313.
74. Pavy B, Iliou MC, Meurin P, et al. Safety of exercise training for cardiac patients: Results of the French registry of complications during cardiac rehabilitation. *Arch Intern Med*. 2006;166:2329–2334.
75. Lavie CJ, Milani RV, Littman AB. Benefits of cardiac rehabilitation and exercise training in secondary coronary prevention in the elderly. *J Am Coll Cardiol*. 1993;22:678–683.
76. Marchionni N, Fattirolli F, Fumagalli S, et al. Improved exercise tolerance and quality of life with cardiac rehabilitation of older patients after myocardial infarction: Results of a randomized, controlled trial. *Circulation*. 2003;107:2201–2206.
77. Frengley JD, Sansone GR, Alba A, Uppal K, Kleinfeld J. Influence of age on rehabilitation outcomes and survival in post-acute inpatient cardiac rehabilitation. *J Cardiopulm Rehabil Prev*. 2011;31:230–238.
78. Parashar S, Spertus JA, Tang F, et al. Predictors of early and late enrollment in cardiac rehabilitation, among those referred, after myocardial infarction. *Circulation*. 2012;126:1587–1595.
79. Balady GJ, Ades PA, Bittner VA, et al. Referral, enrollment, and delivery of cardiac rehabilitation/secondary prevention programs at clinical centers and beyond: A presidential advisory from the American Heart Association. *Circulation*. 2011;124:2951–2960.

80. *National Coverage Determination (NCD) for Cardiac Rehabilitation Programs (20.10)*. Baltimore, MD: Centers for Medicare & Medicaid Services, 2006. Publication No. 100-3. Available at http://www.cms.gov/medicare-coverage-database/details/ncd-details.aspx?NCDId=36&ncdver=2&bc=AgAAQAAAAQAAAA%3d%3d&. Accessed December 14, 2015.
81. Oldridge N, Furlong W, Feeny D, et al. Economic evaluation of cardiac rehabilitation soon after acute myocardial infarction. *Am J Cardiol.* 1993;72:154–161.
82. Taylor R, Kirby B. Cost implications of cardiac rehabilitation in older patients. *Coron Artery Dis.* 1999;10:53–56.
83. Ades PA, Pashkow FJ, Nestor JR. Cost-effectiveness of cardiac rehabilitation after myocardial infarction. *J Cardiopulm Rehabil.* 1997;17:222–231.
84. Goel K, Lennon RJ, Tilbury RT, Squires RW, Thomas RJ. Impact of cardiac rehabilitation on mortality and cardiovascular events after percutaneous coronary intervention in the community. *Circulation.* 2011;123:2344–2352.
85. Pack QR, Goel K, Lahr BD, et al. Participation in cardiac rehabilitation and survival after coronary artery bypass graft surgery: A community-based study. *Circulation.* 2013;128:590–597.
86. *AACVPR Program Directory*. Chicago: American Association of Cardiovascular and Pulmonary Rehabilitation. Available at https://www.aacvpr.org/Resources/Program-Directory. Accessed December 11, 2015.
87. Curnier DY, Savage PD, Ades PA. Geographic distribution of cardiac rehabilitation programs in the United States. *J Cardiopulm Rehabil.* 2005;25:80–84.
88. Brual J, Gravely-Witte S, Suskin N, Stewart DE, Macpherson A, Grace SL. Drive time to cardiac rehabilitation: At what point does it affect utilization? *Int J Health Geogr.* 2010;9:27–38.
89. Shanmugasegaram S, Oh P, Reid RD, McCumber T, Grace SL. A comparison of barriers to use of home- versus site-based cardiac rehabilitation. *J Cardiopulm Rehabil Prev.* 2013;33:297–302.
90. Clark RA, Conway A, Poulsen V, Keech W, Tirimacco R, Tideman P. Alternative models of cardiac rehabilitation: A systematic review. *Eur J Prev Cardiol.* 2015;22:35–74.
91. Clark AM, King-Shier KM, Duncan A, et al. Factors influencing referral to cardiac rehabilitation and secondary prevention programs: A systematic review. *Eur J Prev Cardiol.* 2013;20:692–700.

CHAPTER 11

Secondary Prevention and Lifestyle Modification

Andrew M. Freeman, MD, and Ty J. Gluckman, MD

"Let food be thy medicine and medicine be thy food."
"Walking is man's best medicine."
"Everything in excess is opposed by nature."
–Hippocrates (460 BC – c. 370 BC)

INTRODUCTION

The focus of this book has been on the identification and treatment of patients presenting with acute coronary syndromes (ACSs). As noted in the previous chapter, cardiac rehabilitation is grossly underutilized, leaving practitioners with the responsibility of doing the assessments and facilitating interventions that would have been part of a comprehensive cardiac rehabilitation program. Given the constraints of time available during office visits, it is imperative that practices mobilize their healthcare teams to increase referrals to cardiac rehabilitation and, if not possible or available, have a plan of care for these patients.

Perhaps one of the most important components of ACS care is lifestyle assessment and intervention. Assessment of a patient's risk factors must include an evaluation of their current lifestyle, including diet, exercise, tobacco use, and compliance

Acute Coronary Syndrome: Urgent and Follow-up Care © 2017
Joseph S. Alpert, Lynne T. Braun, Barbara J. Fletcher, Gerald Fletcher, Editors-in-Chief,
Cardiotext Publishing, ISBN: 978-1-935395-94-2

with current medical therapy. It is also important to understand socioeconomic factors such as employment and housing, as well as access to transportation, grocery stores, safe walkable spaces, and other factors that might affect the patient's ability to comply with medical therapy and adopt healthful lifestyle practices. In addition, patients' families and their support system represent key determinants in the success of implementing lifestyle changes and should be factored into the care plan. This assessment can be conducted by the nurse, medical assistant, or other team member so that the healthcare provider can factor in these issues when making recommendations.

Lifestyle modification, while not as sexy as the latest lipid-lowering therapy, is perhaps medicine's oldest and most important intervention. Recently, the world hit a major milestone. There are now more diseases from obesity than from hunger.[1] This revelation is not unexpected in today's world of computers, video games, sedentary lifestyles, fast food, and processed, adulterated food supplies that are readily available at low prices.

While pills undoubtedly work, prevention and attaining goals without medications are often the preferred treatment modalities—but often are not easy for patients to achieve. Every medicine comes with a long list of side effects and potential adverse reactions, but lifestyle modification comes with elbow grease and the need to stay motivated. While adherence to lifestyle modification may be more difficult, many would argue it is the more worthy and lasting approach.

Without healthcare providers sounding the alarm for change, the future of our country, and for that matter the world itself, is headed for an exponential growth in medical expenses, environmental demand that cannot be met, and an enormous burden of disease. Sadly, the average physician has only a few hours of nutrition and exercise didactics or experience, if any at all. As a result, these topics are seldom emphasized in routine clinical encounters.

Modifiable risk factors including dyslipidemia, smoking, hypertension, diabetes mellitus (DM), obesity, an unhealthy diet, and a sedentary lifestyle account for greater than 90% of the population-attributable risk for cardiovascular disease.[2] Furthermore, healthcare providers must act sooner, as elevated cholesterol in early adulthood is associated with cardiovascular disease later in life.[3]

A recent systematic analysis from 199 countries showed that 1.46 billion adults worldwide were estimated to be overweight in 2008, and of these, 502 million were obese.[4] In several studies, obesity accounted for 0.7% to 2.8% of a country's total healthcare costs, and obese individuals cost 30% more than those of normal weight in terms of total healthcare expenditure.[5] In the United States, obesity is estimated to account for 27% of the growth in healthcare expenditure between 1987 and 2001.[6] The annual cost for men with a BMI ≥40 was the equivalent of 1 month of lost productivity and cost employers $3792 per year.[7]

With the projected increase of obesity prevalence in United States adults from about 32% in 2007–2008 (the latest available data) to 50%–51% in 2030 for men (**Figure 11.1**), and from 35% to 45%–52% for women,[8] the United States should expect to see 8 million more cases of diabetes, 6.8 million more cases of coronary heart disease and stroke, and over a half million more cases of cancer over the next 20 years.[9] By 2030, obesity will add $48–$66 billion a year to healthcare costs in the United States and £1.9–£2 billion a year in the UK![9]

Fortunately, there are some efforts to help physicians and patients understand the need for diet, exercise, stress relief, and lifestyle modification. The following example will illustrate how important these efforts will be.

DIET

"Just eat healthy and exercise," says the doctor to his or her patient. Easy, right? Unfortunately, many healthcare providers

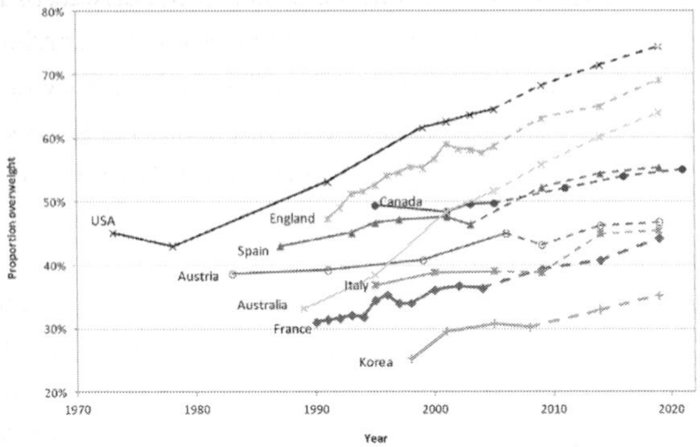

Figure 11.1

Past and projected future proportion of overweight adults. (*Source:* From Franco Sassi. Obesity and the economics of prevention: Fit not fat. Paris: OECD Publishing, 2010. Used with permission.)

do not heed this advice. Providers can often be found squeezing in processed foods between patients, eating business dinners at steakhouses with highly indulgent, rich foods, and not exercising as much as they should.

When healthcare providers do not practice what they preach, or have a deep understanding of what is needed to help their patients, it is difficult for patients to see results and trust what the provider has to say. As such, arming providers with the key dietary knowledge to help their patients (and themselves!) is one of the best ways to succeed. As a provider, when personal transformation occurs, development of the tools and strategies needed to help patients make changes comes more naturally and effortlessly.

Diets are more than restriction of calories. The best way to diet is simply not to diet at all. As is well known, adherence to dieting overall is low and often short-lived.[10] However, when one adopts a lifestyle, and is fully engaged in understanding the pathophysiology of the diseases which come from less-healthy diets, adherence can be increased. Putting patients first and working with them at the center of the care team is a good way to start. Asking about the patient's own barriers to dieting and troubles with weight loss from the past, while appreciating practical issues such as access to fresh produce or budgetary constraints, is a critical first step. Once these factors are considered, outlining a plan for each individual patient should become more straightforward.

Not all diets are equal. While the basic concept of eating fewer calories does lead to weight loss, some diets, particularly those high in plants and low in animal products, may cause additional calories burned by virtue of the type of fuel consumed.[11] Other diets such as Weight Watchers and Nutrisystem, among others, work on restricting portion size. The popular Atkins or Paleo diets focus on consuming little to no carbohydrate and inducing a state of ketogenesis to help achieve weight loss. While no diet is perfect for all, there are some caveats with the high-fat, low-carbohydrate diets. Namely, the red meats and processed animal products that are common staples of these diets are linked to an increased risk of colorectal cancer, heart attack, diabetes, and stroke, even though they can reduce weight and even improve cholesterol temporarily.[12,13] Subjectively, many patients cannot adhere to such a diet for an extended period of time.

A stronger case can be made for plant-based diets. A 100% plant-based diet, which includes a strict vegetarian or vegan diet, has been associated with 1) improved cardiovascular outcomes, 2) decreased cancer risk,[14,15] and 3) improvement or elimination of DM.[16] This type of diet, along with exercise, is perhaps one of the most powerful tools to reduce cardiovascular disease,[17] but is underutilized. Importantly, this is not a diet solely of salads—but a diet rich in whole grains, legumes, tubers, vegetables, seeds, nuts, and fruits.

Getting a patient to change long-ingrained, conditioned patterns is challenging. For some, a primary cardiac event is a "wakeup call," but many do not adhere long term. One example that can be reinforced is the fact that most stenting procedures do not save lives, but rather alleviate symptoms[18] and help patients buy time to make the lifestyle changes they need to reduce their future risk. Sharing this information is often one of the key educational "aha" moments that a provider is obliged to do. Once a patient understands that stents and modern medicine only fix one part of a systemic disease process, the buy-in increases.

A critical way to engage patients is to provide internet-based and printed materials that educate patients about healthier eating. Some examples are listed in **Table 11.1**. A thorough understanding of the data behind this type of diet and real-world solutions is key. For example, one of the many questions heard includes "Can I eat out?" The answer is, of course, an emphatic yes. Eating out requires careful planning; however, by researching the menus ahead of time, is easy to do. For instance, one can have pizza, but the goal is to avoid the cheese and meat. While this may seem like heresy in our cheese-loving society, in Italy, this is commonly eaten and is known as "tomato pie." With a good sauce, some freshly sautéed vegetables, and good seasoning, this will quickly become a favorite for many at Italian restaurants. Or, at a Mexican restaurant, one might enjoy brown rice with veggies and salsa, without the need for meat, cheese, and sour cream. For those on a budget, brown rice and beans are quick, inexpensive, thoroughly nutritious, and satiating. There are several documentary movies on these topics that are inspirational, and can help to motivate patients to make significant changes.

One of the best tools to engage patients is the care team that includes advanced practice providers, registered dieticians, and nutritionists. Having patients meet with these providers one-on-one to tailor a diet and lifestyle plan with close monitoring can be very effective at producing better outcomes.

Table 11.1
A Listing of Selected Websites to Empower your Patients to Learn to Eat Well

http://www.pcrm.org	Physicians Committee for Responsible Medicine: A great resource for getting people to understand how to be plant-based eaters. Includes a Vegetarian Starter Kit
http://www.cardiosmart.org/Healthy-Living/Eat-Better	CardioSmart.org: The American College of Cardiology's guide to eating better
http://ohsheglows.com	A blog by one of the more outspoken vegan cooks which shows folks how to eat more plant-based
http://www.aarp.org/health/healthy-living/info-08-2013/bill-clinton-vegan.html	AARP shows how former President Bill Clinton goes vegan
http://www.forksoverknives.com	Forks Over Knives: A documentary on why eating plant-based foods can change lives and also has associated cookbooks
http://www.nativefoods.com	An example of a restaurant chain, native foods, which is 100% plant-based
http://www.webmd.com/diet/features/skinny-diet-not-big-on-meatw-sweets	WebMD's discussion of eating Skinny Vegan
http://www.drfuhrman.com	Dr. Furhman's work on eating plant-based foods
http://www.thechinastudy.com	The China Study: The work of Dr. T. Colin Campbell and his studies of nutrition worldwide
http://www.hungryforchange.tv	Hungry For Change: A documentary about eating well
http://www.nutritionaction.org	Nutrition Action: A monthly newsletter explains the hidden dangers of commonly consumed foods

EXERCISE

Using exercise as medicine is a difficult concept to convey to patients. While medicine can be effective at controlling symptoms, it rarely cures disease. With medications, there are often side-effects that can compromise compliance and prevent long-lasting effects. Balancing this with exercise and a healthy lifestyle, however, *can* cure disease. Sharing these pearls of wisdom often has them ask the question of how they might improve or avoid a second cardiovascular event without the need for more medication.

Fortunately, exercise has been shown to lower blood pressure, improve cholesterol, reduce diastolic dysfunction, decrease the likelihood of developing cancer, and improve longevity.[19–21] The only problem is getting your patients to actually do this. Most physicians never discuss this time-tested, proven "medicine" with their patients—and this needs to change. Just 30 minutes a day is what the American Heart Association (AHA) suggests is enough to see significant effects. For the average person, this means 23.5 hours every day is free to do whatever one pleases, but at least 30 minutes should be dedicated to this effort.

Some have shown promise with the exercise prescription (**Figure 11.2**). A provider simply lists the amount of time needed for exercise and writes it as if it were a medicine. The prescription serves as a reminder to patients on just how important this type of activity is for well-being. Some research suggests that the exercise prescription with written support materials is an effective way to boost compliance.[22]

Human beings were designed to move and be active. As such, activity during the day that's either part of work or related to self-care is good, but not good enough. In addition, just "hitting the gym" with weightlifting falls short. When one exercises for health, the absolute heart rate or caloric expenditure is not as important as the individual finding his or her own fitness level and needs. As such, working to a level that makes one unable to verbally complete a sentence, sweating if warm enough, and dyspneic is critical.

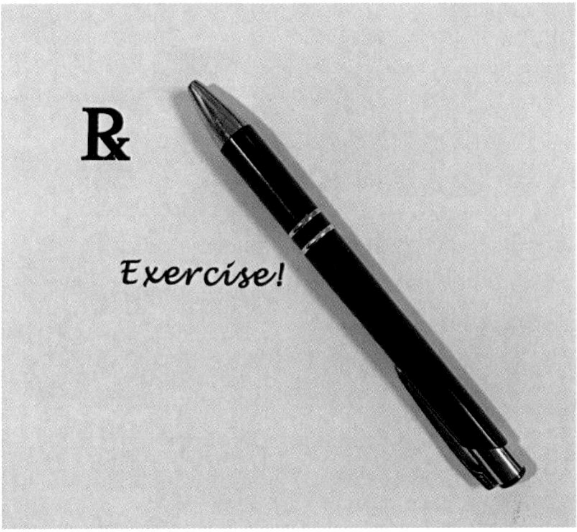

Figure 11.2

Research suggests that a written exercise prescription with support materials is an effective tool to boost compliance.

Many of your patients will tell you that they cannot do this. For these individuals, enrollment in cardiac or pulmonary rehabilitation is a good starting point, but this is not and should not be the limit of one's exercise. Familiarity with different exercise modalities will make regular activity more natural. For many patients, an assistive device such as a walker with a seat is very helpful. Such a device allows a patient to work to a challenging workload, but rest anytime the need arises. It also allows quick resumption of activity. When a patient is first starting to incorporate these activities, it may take 60, 90, or even 120 minutes to perform 30 minutes of good brisk activities. The goal should be to work on reducing the break times as the weeks go on.

The average human walking speed is 3 mi/h. Most folks walk briskly at 4 mi/h and start jogging at 5 mi/h. Using the "breath test," which is the point at which one becomes unable to complete a sentence while exercising, most patients should aim to cover 2 miles in 30 minutes or 4 mi/h. For those who cannot walk, other means of cardiovascular activity are acceptable, but there is an important caveat: machines, bicycles, and conveyance equipment of any sort is designed to optimize distance and reduce effort. As such, on a bicycle, for example, one should put enough resistance on the wheel so that when the participant stops movement, so does the machine.

Group effort always produces better results. As such, individuals should seek out local community efforts that may be helpful. In many cities, there are national Walk with a Doc chapters (http://www.walkwithadoc.org), with other such programs worldwide. With this program, physicians participate in walks, usually outside in parks, side-by-side with patients in an effort to "walk the walk" and "practice what is preached." Coupled with healthy snacks and a talk by a local expert physician, these walks empower people to do more, be part of a group, and use the power of social networks to encourage regular exercise outside of these walks. These walks engage local physicians, nurses, exercise physiologists, and dieticians to walk with patients and answer questions in a relaxed atmosphere. This helps to remove traditional barriers to care while providing much needed education, combined with the power of walking.

Including your physical therapy team, advanced practice providers, and nurses in exercise planning only helps to reinforce the importance of this approach. Exercise is free, highly effective, and has better outcomes than most pills, with the only side effect being the need for motivation and effort. It can be done anywhere at anytime, and when combined with diet and stress relief should be a first-line therapy for cardiovascular protection and disease prevention.

STRESS RELIEF

Stress from everyday life is unavoidable. Living in the modern world creates stress from relationships, work environments, finances, daily decisions, illness and more. Patients who suffer heart attacks are much more likely to be depressed and subsequently suffer from significant amounts of stress.[23] As such, mindful activity is critical to being able to decompress from daily stress.

Stress relief takes many forms, but is not simply talking out one's problems. In fact, many patients do best with introspective time or by doing activities by themselves that are unrelated to work, business, or family. Some patients work on meditation or simply spend time listening to their breathing. Others take on hobbies, crafts, or work outside the home such as gardening. Whatever form is taken, stress-relieving activities help reduce disease (sometimes spelled dis-ease to emphasize the concept of disease being from lack of ease, i.e., stress) and the likelihood of adverse outcomes. Still others require professional counseling to effectively lessen the impact of stress.

Stress has been shown to increase the risk of heart attack,[24] as has an angry attitude.[25] Stress has also been shown to increase cholesterol, and often can manifest as palpitations and chest pain. The physical toll of emotional stress can sometimes be overwhelming.

Unfortunately, providers spend little time talking about mental health and stress-relieving activities. They often do not realize, themselves, just how important mental well-being can be to health. As such, patients should be coached to give themselves 30 minutes of stress-relieving activities each day. This time, combined with 30 minutes of walking, should be treated as a nearly sacred "power hour" which serves to promote health and create a state of mental well-being. Many who exercise have experienced this combination of physical work and mental relaxation, commonly referred to as the "runner's high." This type of feeling and effort can go far to improve health and should be implemented side-by-side with diet for maximum effect. Obviously, significant stress, bereavement, or mental illness should be evaluated by a qualified mental health professional.

PUTTING IT ALL TOGETHER

This section has attempted to illustrate the power of medicine's most basic and simple tool—lifestyle modification—in the reduction of future risk for ACS patients. Through the effects of a plant-based, whole food, unprocessed diet, coupled with exercise and mindfulness/stress relief, health can be maintained and even restored in many cases.

While it may be impossible to conduct a study to purely test the outcomes of these interventions, there are more than enough good data to support widespread adoption of these measures. In an era where polypharmacy is often treated as the solution to disease, it is nice to know that disease can be halted by alternative, low-cost measures which are attainable and widely available.

A lifestyle similar to that of many ancient and rural cultures has demonstrated enormous wisdom: eat what grows, limit processed foods and animal products, exercise religiously and work hard, and spend time in introspection and with friends and family. Combining these items in today's high-technology, sedentary world can have enormous impact on our future.

In summary, it is eminently possible to change the future risk for ACS patients, by utilizing all members of the healthcare team (with the right staff person in the right role) to assess patients, provide education and support for lifestyle changes, and maintain constant reinforcement.

REFERENCES

1. Lozano R, Naghavi M, Foreman K, et al. Global and regional mortality from 235 causes of death for 20 age groups in 1990 and 2010: A systematic analysis for the Global Burden of Disease Study 2010. *Lancet*. 2012;380(9859):2095–2128.

2. *Global Atlas on Cardiovascular Disease Prevention and Control.* Mendis S, Puska P, Norrving B, Eds. Geneva: World Health Organization. 2011.
3. Pearson TA, LaCroix AZ, Mead LA, Liang KY. The prediction of midlife coronary heart disease and hypertension in young adults: The Johns Hopkins multiple risk equations. *Am J Prev Med.* 1990; 6(2 Suppl):23–28.
4. Finucane MM, Stevens GA, Cowan MJ, et al. National, regional, and global trends in body-mass index since 1980: Systematic analysis of health examination surveys and epidemiological studies with 960 country-years and 9.1 million participants. *Lancet.* 2011;377:557–567.
5. Withrow D, Alter DA. The economic burden of obesity worldwide: A systematic review of the direct costs of obesity. *Obes Rev.* 2011;12:131–141.
6. Thorpe KE, Florence CS, Howard DH, Joski P. The impact of obesity on rising medical spending. *Health Aff (Millwood).* Jul-Dec 2004;Suppl Web Exclusives:W4-480–W4-486.
7. Finkelstein EA, DiBonaventura MD, Burgess SM, Hale BC. The costs of obesity in the workplace. *J Occup Environ Med.* 2010;52:971–976.
8. Wang Y, Beydoun MA, Liang L, Caballero B, Kumanyika SK. Will all Americans become overweight or obese? Estimating the progression and cost of the U.S. obesity epidemic. *Obesity (Silver Spring).* 2008;16:2323–2330.
9. Wang Y, McPherson K, Marsh T, Gortmaker SL, Brown M. Health and economic burden of the projected obesity trends in the USA and the UK. *Lancet.* 2011;378:815–825.
10. Larsen TM, Dalskov SM, van Baak M, et al. Diets with high or low protein content and glycemic index for weight-loss maintenance. *N Engl J Med.* 2010;363(22):2102–2113.
11. Mishra S, Xu J, Agarwal U, Gonzales J, Levin S, Barnard ND. A multicenter randomized controlled trial of a plant-based nutrition program to reduce body weight and cardiovascular risk in the corporate setting: The GEICO study. *Eur J Clin Nutr.* 2013;67:718–724.
12. Pan A, Sun Q, Bernstein AM, et al. Red meat consumption and mortality: Results from 2 prospective cohort studies. *Arch Intern Med.* 2012;172:555–563.
13. Pan A, Sun Q, Bernstein AM, Manson JE, Willett WC, Hu FB. Changes in red meat consumption and subsequent risk of type 2 diabetes mellitus: Three cohorts of U.S. men and women. *JAMA Intern Med.* 2013;173:1328–1335.
14. Ornish D, Scherwitz LW, Billings JH, et al. Intensive lifestyle changes for reversal of coronary heart disease. *JAMA.* 1998;280:2001–2007.
15. Ornish D, Weidner G, Fair WR, et al. Intensive lifestyle changes may affect the progression of prostate cancer. *J Urol.* 2005;174:1065–1069.

16. Silberman A, Banthia R, Estay IS, et al. The effectiveness and efficacy of an intensive cardiac rehabilitation program in 24 sites. *Am J Health Promot*. 2010;24:260–266.
17. Ornish D, Brown SE, Scherwitz LW, et al. Can lifestyle changes reverse coronary heart disease? The Lifestyle Heart Trial. *Lancet*. 1990;336:129–133.
18. Boden WE, O'Rourke RA, Teo KK, et al. Optimal medical therapy with or without PCI for stable coronary disease. *N Engl J Med*. 2007;356:1503–1516.
19. Wen CP, Wai JP, Tsai MK, et al. Minimum amount of physical activity for reduced mortality and extended life expectancy: A prospective cohort study. *Lancet*. 2011;378:1244–1253.
20. Bourque JM, Hollan BH, Watson DD, Beller GA. Achieving an exercise workload of ≥10 metabolic equivalents predicts a very low risk of inducible ischemia: Does myocardial perfusion imaging have a role? *J Am Coll Cardiol*. 2009;54:538–545.
21. Chomistek A. Vigorous physical activity, mediating biomarkers, and risk of myocardial infarction. *Med Sci Sports Exerc*. 2011;43:1884–1890.
22. Smith BJ, Bauman AE, Bull FC, Booth ML, Harris MF. Promoting physical activity in general practice: A controlled trial of written advice and information materials. *Br J Sports Med*. 2000;34:262–267.
23. Vögele C, Christ O, Spaderna H. Cardiac threat appraisal and depression after first myocardial infarction. *Front Psychol*. 2012;3:365.
24. Nabi H, Kivimäki M, Batty GD, et al. Increased risk of coronary heart disease among individuals reporting adverse impact of stress on their health: The Whitehall II prospective cohort study. *Eur Heart J*. 2013;34:2697–2705.
25. Kawachi I, Sparrow D, Spiro A, III, Vokonas P, Weiss ST. A prospective study of anger and coronary heart disease. The Normative Aging Study. *Circulation*. 1996;94:2090–2095.

Index

Page numbers followed by *f*, *t*, refer to figures, tables.

D

H

I

K

L

M

N